D1461264

ENCOURAGING DIVERSITY:
VOLUNTARY AND PRIVATE ORGANISATIONS
IN COMMUNITY CARE

Encouraging Diversity: Voluntary and Private Organisations in Community Care

Marilyn Taylor
Joan Langan
Paul Hoggett

School for Advanced Urban Studies
University of Bristol

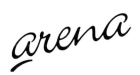

© Marilyn Taylor, Joan Langan, Paul Hoggett 1995

All rights reserved. No part of this publication may be reproduced, stored in a retrieval system, or transmitted in any form or by any means, electronic, mechanical, photocopying, recording or otherwise without the prior permission of the publisher.

Published by
Arena
Ashgate Publishing Limited
Gower House
Croft Road
Aldershot
Hants GU11 3HR
England

Ashgate Publishing Company
Old Post Road
Brookfield
Vermont 05036
USA

British Library Cataloguing in Publication Data

Taylor, Marilyn
   Encouraging Diversity: Voluntary and
   Private Organisations in Community Care
   I. Title
   361.7630941

1 85742 281 3

Library of Congress Catalog Card Number: 94–79820

The Joseph Rowntree Foundation has supported this project as part of its programme of research and innovative development projects, which it hopes will be of value to policy makers and practitioners. The facts presented and views expressed in this report, however, are those of the authors and not necessarily those of the Foundation.

Some of the information contained in this report can also be found in: Dallago, B. and Mittone, L. (eds) (forthcoming) *Economic Institutions, Markets and Competition: Centralization and decentralization in the transformation of economic systems*, Aldershot: Edward Elgar.

Typeset in 12 point Palatino by Raven Typesetters, Chester
Printed and bound in Great Britain by
Biddles Limited, Guildford and King's Lynn

Contents

Acknowledgements

Many people have been involved in the writing of this report. We are particularly grateful for the time and support given to us by our 33 case study organisations and by other people from our three localities who shared their time and their observations with us. It goes without saying that, without them, the report could not have been written. Thanks are also due to the Joseph Rowntree Foundation, both for their financial support and for the encouragement and advice given to us as the study developed. Our national advisory committee and the local advisory groups in areas B and C provided many useful comments as the work progressed and we are grateful for their time and expertise. We would also like to thank Jenny Capstick, Lorraine Cantle, Mark Cox, Valerie Douglas and Katharine Green for computing and administrative support. Finally, thanks are due to our partners, families and friends, who gave us encouragement and support when we needed it.

Marilyn Taylor
Joan Langan
Paul Hoggett

August 1994

1
Introduction

Background

Community care services have been subject to radical changes in recent years. These changes, enshrined in the NHS and Community Care Act 1990, reflect a belief that the transfer of much of the delivery of service to non-statutory providers will be more efficient and cost-effective than the public welfare bureaucracies of the past. Non-statutory services are seen as likely to be more responsive and provide greater choice to service users and carers than over-standardised and dependency-creating public services.

Choice ultimately depends on the user's right to a service and on their control over decisions as to what kind of service they will get. Until they have that right, the display of goods and services on offer is a secondary consideration. But, that said, a wide diversity of service providers should allow for greater choice and provide the opportunity for innovation, flexibility and different patterns of care. It should also increase the resources on which society can call in meeting its community care needs.

The community care reforms mean that statutory authorities now have responsibilities to support and stimulate the market so that the range of services available reflects need more closely. Efficiency and choice are to be promoted through importing market principles such as competition and contracting into the provision of community care. But while the principle of greater diversity and choice is welcomed by voluntary and private organisations, many commentators have expressed concern about the changes. Some question the appropriateness of market principles to the provision of a public service whose effectiveness relies on continuity and the quality of relationships (Leat, 1993b). Others doubt whether the diversity that the reforms intend will be achieved against a background of expenditure cuts. Financial pressures could mean increasing reliance upon care provided at the margins of the labour force. There are fears, too, that the values and distinctiveness of agencies in the non-statutory sectors may be undermined and that their diversity may suffer, as smaller agencies or those providing activities which are not a priority for new statutory purchasing policies find it increasingly hard to survive.

If new policies are to offer real choices to service users, to release resources and use them effectively, it is essential that policy makers and purchasers understand the diversity and complexity of the organisations on which they are calling. It is also important for non-statutory organisations themselves to get a sense of how they fit into the total pattern of provision and to have confidence in their distinctive contribution – to 'position' themselves in the new market.

The research

The study reported here maps private and voluntary organisations providing community care services (Chapter 2). It explores the values and motivations which drive them, the way in which they are structured and managed in order to put these values into practice and the implications for those using the services (Chapters 3 and 4). It also asks how new demands and new policies are affecting their ability to deliver their services (Chapter 5). Most importantly of all, it asks whether the community care reforms will increase the range of choices available to service users and carers.

The study draws on information from three localities, urban, suburban and rural, chosen to reflect different political traditions along a spectrum from market-orientated to state-orientated (see Appendix B). Information was gathered through a postal survey, local interviews to establish patterns of provision and case studies based on interviews with 33 organisations, with four carried out over a number of visits (details of the research methodology can be found in Appendix A).

The findings

This book is not about choosing between organisations in this new policy environment. It does not set out to find a 'best buy' for the community care purchaser. Its focus is on diversity: how far it already exists; what it offers; and how it can be developed, sustained and strengthened into the future. It questions traditional assumptions about the different sectors in community care, suggesting that size and whether an organisation is run by or for users may be just as important in making sense of the diversity that exists as whether it is private or voluntary. It stresses the interdependence between organisations, whether from the public, voluntary or private sectors, and the networks of support and care on which service users and carers depend. It identifies increasing pressures away from diversity and towards growth, formalisation and growing similarity between organisations, pressures which are reinforced by current management values and the implementation of policy.

In the face of these pressures, in Chapter 6, it makes a number of recommendations to government, both local and central, as to how diversity can be fostered and sustained. These are:

Local and health authorities need to:
- Maintain an up-to-date picture of their local voluntary and private sectors – who is out there, what they provide, how they operate and where they fit into local patterns of provision.
- Invest in development – provide the core funds and infrastructure which will allow organisations to respond to new demands and needs and maintain their long-term viability.
- Invest in variety – have a variety of funding arrangements so that small and new organisations can benefit as well as larger and better-known organisations; continue to invest in the patchwork of 'taken-for-granted' services and activities which prevent crisis and support priority services.
- Invest in advocacy – informed choices depend on information and advocacy, while effective and informed consultation depends on those who are consulted having the resources and encouragement to develop a confident contribution.
- Find a balance between the need to ensure quality and safety and levels of regulation which stifle creativity and responsiveness; invest in user- and carer-led organisations to help them define the standards they want from service providers.
- Recognise the importance of networks within and between sectors and support their development. They can be especially crucial to the survival of small, locally-based agencies.

Central government needs to:
- Recognise the need for long-term investment if a truly mixed economy of care is to develop, and support purchasing authorities in making the investments we recommend.

- Recognise the need for local authorities to maintain their own provision, even if on a more limited and competitive basis than in the past.
- Explore the possibility of adapting charity law to allow user-based organisations to benefit from tax privileges, to ensure that service users and community representatives are not deterred from involvement as trustees, and to allow autonomy for local branches where appropriate.

2
Mapping the territory

The organisations we found across the three localities in the study demonstrate the diversity of provision that already exists in the voluntary and private sectors. They ranged from: community centres run by minority ethnic groups and offering a wide variety of services, to small residential homes for elderly people; small voluntary visiting services and clubs to a large corporate care firm; advocacy services run by ex-service users to a professional counselling agency; private home care agencies run by one person to a trust of 18 'floated-off' local authority homes. Some of these organisations already provide the mainstream services that current policy wishes to see transferred to independent organisations. Others provide services and support that can prevent crisis and reduce pressure on mainstream and crisis provision. They do this by giving people more confidence in themselves, someone to turn to for help and advice, a roof over their heads, a way out of isolation and loneliness or counselling to build on periods of more intensive care. Many voluntary organisations are involved in public education and campaigning as well as service provision, to increase government and public understanding of the needs they were set up to meet and to inform the public policy process.

Central government tends to use the term 'independent

sector' to describe this diversity, while common usage distinguishes between the 'private' and 'voluntary sectors'. However, the idea of 'sector' is more and more inadequate to the task of describing the range of organisations that can be found in the expanding world outside the public sector. New groups run by service users stress the fact that they are different from the traditional concept of the voluntary sector as one which helps others. The term 'not-for-profit' is increasingly being used to describe a territory somewhere between voluntary, as traditionally understood, and private. Several commentators have suggested that differences of size and degree of organisation *within* sectors may be as important as those *between* them (Paton, 1992; Billis, 1993; Knight, 1993; Leat, 1993a). Private agencies in our study stressed the difference between small family firms and partnerships, on the one hand, and large corporate concerns with shareholders. A network of private sector providers in one of the localities we studied specifically excluded the corporate sector.

To reflect this and building on work by Paton (1992), we built a new organisational map, based on two dimensions: ownership and complexity (see Fig. 1).

Ownership

The idea of 'ownership' retains the distinction between private and voluntary but divides the voluntary sector[1] into three, according to whether an organisation is run on a mutual basis ('by us for us') or for the benefit of others ('by them for us'). Thus, to the category of private, are added:

1. In the rest of the report, the term 'voluntary sector' is used when talking collectively of user, community and donor organisations, while 'independent sector' is used to cover all voluntary and private organisations.

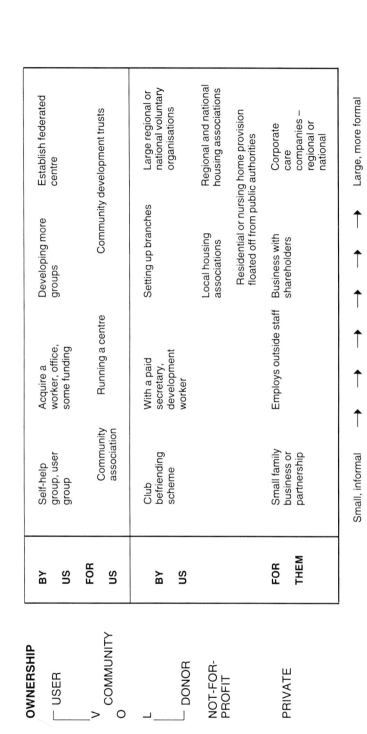

Figure 1   Ownership and complexity

- **community** (run by and for people from a particular neighbourhood, or a minority ethnic community);
- **user** (run by service users or ex-users, or by carers for carers[2]);
- **donor** (where people give their time or money to help others).

Housing associations emerged from our questionnaires as a separate not-for-profit category to which we added trusts and companies 'floated off' from public authorities. Although we only had two within our sample, we would expect to see a rapid increase in trusts formed to 'float off' public services. There is already an umbrella body formed to represent their interests.

One further category which we mention for the sake of completeness, but which did not appear in our study, is that of staff-owned organisations and co-operatives. The lack of co-operatives in our study is partly a reflection of political and cultural traditions – the co-operative tradition is weak in the UK compared with, for example, southern Europe (but see Spear et al., 1994).

Degree of complexity

This places organisations along a continuum. At one end are small, highly-integrated organisations with few 'stakeholders' where the people who decide policy and manage are the people who do the work and provide the major resources. At the other are large, complex organisations where policy formulation is separated from management, operations and funding.

2. References in the report to user organisations will include organisations run by carers for carers, i.e. where carers themselves are the users of the services and support they provide.

This map is not static – as the diagram shows, organisations may move from one part to another as they grow and change. But from the questionnaire survey, it was possible to draw up the following profiles for the main types of organisation we found. We then drew our 33 case studies from across this organisational map. Descriptions of the case study organisations are given in Appendix C, while further details of the questionnaire responses are given in Appendix D.

User
(40) These organisations concentrated upon the provision of leisure, social activities, support, counselling, advocacy or campaigning activities. They were membership-based organisations with smaller and simpler management committees than any other organisation within the voluntary sector. Their management committees were usually elected rather than appointed. Our survey suggested that fewer than one in four had a budget greater than £5,000 per annum or received any form of grant aid.

Donor

i) simple   (33) These organisations tended to focus on the provision of social and support services. They were more likely to be formally constituted than user organisations, typically as a charitable trust. However, like user organisations, the majority generated their small income from donations, fundraising and subscriptions. They tended to operate at the very local level, i.e. the neighbourhood, whereas user organisations were as likely to operate at the level of a town, city or county as at the neighbourhood level.

ii) complex   (44 non-residential, 28 residential) Such organisations provided a wider range of services to a broader range of clients across more extensive catchment areas than any other type of organisation. They had the largest and most complex management committees (in terms of the variety of interests represented) and were more likely to have user representatives on the management committee than simple donors, especially if they provided non-residential services. They relied upon the most diverse range of funding sources.

Not-for-profit
(32) The housing associations in our study were more likely to serve elderly people than other groups and to cover an area larger than the immediate locality. Two out of three were constituted as Industrial and Provident Associations. Nearly half had users on their management committee. They all had paid staff and all but two had incomes over £100,000, which came from central government (via the Housing Corporation) or fees. The other two not-for-profits were two trusts formed by public authorities to 'float off' either statutory residential or nursing home provision.

Private organisations
(66) The private sector organisations we surveyed offered three main kinds of service – domiciliary care and home nursing, general nursing care, or residential and nursing home care – nearly always to elderly people. They were more likely to be stand-alone organisations than others in the sample and had a simpler management structure: with the exception of the seven corporate companies who responded to the survey, most were owner-managed (three out of four) or had boards of no more than three members. They were younger than the other organisations who responded to our survey: four out of five were formed since 1979, compared to only half of other organisations. Three

out of four derived at least some of their income from state benefits. Of particular interest is the fact that one in four used volunteers, although in most cases, the number cited was no more than four.

Community organisations
(9) These were surveyed in only one locality, in order to ensure coverage of organisations in ethnic minority communities there, since more specialist organisations were relatively undeveloped for these groups.

Voluntary residential homes had the oldest age profile of any organisation in our sample – almost as many were formed before 1960 as after 1979. This contrasts strongly with the much younger privately-run residential and nursing homes. Over recent years, it has been in the residential sector that most opportunities have been created for the private sector to take over from the statutory sector. Indeed private residential homes were more likely than any other group to have been formed since 1979. Housing associations were most likely to have been formed between 1960 and 1979.

3
Values and motivation

The assumption is frequently made that private organisations have different values from voluntary organisations and are more likely to be driven by profit. This chapter examines the values found within organisations in the study and their implications for service users.

Values

We found a range of values[1] across the organisations we studied.

Caring for others   philanthropy, family and spiritual values:

'love of older people'
'to help those less fortunate'
'doing what any family member would do'
'all one happy family'
'do as you would have done unto you'.

---

1. In our study we relied on people's descriptions of their organisation's values. We did not evaluate how far they were put into practice. However, we did gather information from people in different parts of the organisation.

Promoting independence   giving people privacy within a residential setting or keeping them in their own home:

   'privacy and dignity'
   'space for residents to live as independently as possible';

developmental approaches, including normalisation and therapy:

   'to support people in living independent lives, support rather than care'.

Market consumerism   emphasising the physical quality of the service and the rights of the paying consumer:

   'serving the customer: they pay so they come first'
   'the residents are our customers and if they want hotel-style care, they should get it'
   'we want to be the Marks and Spencer of community care'.

Mutuality   support among people working together from a common experience, reinforcing common identity:

   'our own place to discuss problems and socialise'.

Empowerment   seeking to change the nature of services which marginalise communities and disable users, and give users an individual and collective 'voice':

   'supporting people to have their own voice'
   'access to what other people get'
   'sheer bloody-mindedness. We think we've got a point to make'
   'equality; civil rights'.

Caring values could be found across our organisational map and were particularly common in organisations serving older people. Spiritual values were also found across the map: in a private residential home which the owners had bought when the charitable trust they worked for was wound up; a medical mission which was now a charity running residential homes; a minority ethnic community organisation; and a housing association which had grown from a religious discussion group. Development values like normalisation and therapy were reported by professional staff in both private and donor organisations. They were most likely to be found in organisations for people with learning difficulties and mental health problems, but rare among organisations serving elderly people. Some respondents commented on the lack of positive models for this care group. Market consumerism was most likely to be found in private organisations. Mutuality and empowerment, on the other hand, were not reported as values in private organisations and were most common in community and user organisations.

Different values were found in the same organisation, especially in larger organisations or organisations with several different activities. Community organisations in our sample were concerned with caring and providing a family atmosphere for elders as well as empowerment and mutuality for the community at large. An organisation with a number of projects under its umbrella reported that these encompassed a range of different goals and values. Different values were also found at different levels in an organisation: philanthropy and caring among trustees, for example, or consumerism among managers of private agencies, development among professional staff, family values among non-professional staff and volunteers, empowerment among users and so on.

User control

User and community organisations were often explicitly concerned with giving users and members of marginalised communities control over their own services and a collective voice in the planning and delivery of services provided by others.

> *Two years ago, I couldn't have done this. I can do things here I can't do anywhere else* (user volunteer in a user organisation).

For the private sector, the contract with their customers meant that their wishes had to be pre-eminent: 'They have total control. It's what they want. We can make suggestions.' Service users could always take their custom elsewhere if they did not like the service on offer. This form of control could be very empowering for those where money was no object or who could 'shop around' for another provider (this is easier in home care than in residential care). But it excludes those who do not have access to either private or public funds and is difficult to exercise where continuity of support is crucial.

Organisations whose predominant values were caring, whether from the private, donor or community sectors, emphasised their role in freeing the individual user from care or giving them opportunities (e.g. to get out of the house) that they had not had before. It is certainly true that, until people's basic needs are met, any other kind of empowerment is unlikely (Maslow, 1943). Some professionals in these organisations saw their role as empowering users by developing their capacity to gain control over their own lives and take risks. Approaches such as normalisation, counselling and other therapies belonged in this category.

User organisations argued that caring could be patronising and disempowering. They were also critical of professional developmental approaches, such as normalisation, as imposing external values of what is normal on disabled people.

A number of respondents stressed the need to allow service users to choose whether they were 'developed' and 'involved' or not. Some users said they didn't want to be forced to engage in activities and didn't find user meetings helpful. Several agencies spoke of the tension between a desire to encourage people to reach their potential and the need to ensure that the choice was theirs: 'People may not want to change, even if the carer thinks they should'. One key lesson from this study is that the range of services on offer should allow people the choice to be involved in different ways. User-based advocacy organisations can help them make this choice.

The significance of profit

Economists have argued that profit is essential to the effective operation of a market in community care, as an incentive to new providers (Le Grand and Bartlett, 1993). It is often assumed that, in the private sector, considerations of profit will outweigh other values, and that voluntary agencies are more 'trustworthy', a view that was shared by many voluntary organisations in our study and by at least one of the statutory authorities.

We found, however, that this view of the differences between the sectors was too simple. Respondents from two of the larger private agencies did report their first priority as making a profit and in the two corporate care firms we studied managers did have profitability targets to reach. But, while profit is always a consideration, caring and family values were also evident in all the private agencies we studied, while some staff subscribed to developmental values emphasising the autonomy and dignity of residents. One private agency had been prepared to cut profit margins to improve quality and to leave a bed empty, with the loss of revenue that represented, in order to ensure new residents fitted in with the existing group. Several owners or managers of small private homes or home care agencies in our study put in long hours – indeed this was the only way some of them could survive financially. If profit was the only consideration, we would have expected them to fold.

Several private organisations were set up by people who had worked in the public sector and employed people trained in the public or voluntary sectors, who had brought 'public sector values' with them. There seemed to be a number of motivations that drove these people into the private sector. Several now saw the private sector as the best way of meeting a need they identified because it gave them the opportunity to be their own boss, to get away from the bureaucracy which they saw in the statutory sector, to be independent and flexible. These motivations are comparable with those described elsewhere as belonging to 'craftsmen entrepreneurs' in contrast to 'opportunistic entrepreneurs', whose primary motivation is not capital accumulation (Marceau, 1990; Taylor and Hoggett, 1994).

Even where profit is a major consideration for owners, shareholders and managers, the front-line staff we interviewed in for-profit agencies were often motivated by very similar values to front-line staff in other sectors: many worked in the private sector because that's where they were able to find a job; some said that although they had reservations about working for a private agency before they started, they had not found that these were justified. This view was echoed by relatives of residents in two of the agencies we studied.

It is still possible that caring and developmental values

are more common in voluntary than private organisations – our study did not put this to the test. The number of private agencies among our case studies was small (eight) and it is possible to argue that only the most 'public-spirited' replied to our questionnaire. For example, two of the agencies we studied were reported to be above average for the private sector with respect to terms and conditions for their staff – both also gave workers access to training and qualifications as a matter of policy.

Certainly, even those in the private sector had reservations about others from their sector and gave examples of agencies who were only interested in the bottom line, who exploited staff, who charged for everything other than absolute necessities or where the owner only set foot in the door to demand further cuts in costs. One carer said of the home where her father had previously lived that: 'You can see the money signs in their eyes.' A respondent from a user organisation who had worked with residents in private homes estimated that terms and conditions there were generally below average (for research reinforcing this impression, see Bland, 1993), leading to high turnover and extensive use of agency staff. This is not likely to deliver continuity of care.

Nonetheless, some respondents thought the days when smaller operators could make a big profit had gone with the end of the property boom and the financial reforms in community care. If so, the individual owner who wanted to make a quick profit would no longer see this as an attractive area in which to set up a business. The real danger to caring values, according to some of the private organisations we studied, now lay with the entry into the caring market of big corporate firms from other sectors of the economy – breweries, construction companies and insurance companies were mentioned. There was some concern that the motivation of large care companies seeking to improve their profit margins was likely to be different from that of smaller home-owners. One of the authorities in the study received bids from a number of industrial cleaning companies when it put a home care operation out to tender. It had rejected these out of hand, but there is no guarantee that, as financial constraints continue to bite, this discrimination will continue into the future.

We did not carry out a systematic comparison of values and practice between the sectors. The most we can say is that there is likely to be 'good' and 'bad' in all types of organisations. However, if they want to compete effectively in new markets, it seems that voluntary agencies will need to establish their distinctiveness from the private sector in terms other than a claim to superior values. If profit crowds out all other considerations in a private agency, then the quality of service is likely to suffer. But there is nothing wrong with profit *per se* and in a situation where voluntary organisations themselves are expected to develop marketing strategies and develop a healthy 'bottom line', it may be hard for purchasers to see a difference.

There seemed to us to be two very clear value differences between private (and some not-for-profit) agencies and voluntary organisations. Mutuality and collective empowerment values were not expressed by private organisations, none of whom were engaged in campaigning for their service users. Not-for-profits, too, were less likely to engage in 'political' activity – indeed one 'floated-off' trust said it did not consider itself a voluntary organisation because it did not campaign.

We observed two further differences. Two respondents felt that there was less protection for continuity of values in private organisations if ownership changed than there was under charitable law. One not-for-profit trust was concerned about the possible implications when the freehold of its properties, previously held by the health authority, was put out to tender. However, while this protection may be provided by charitable law in theory, trust deeds can still provide considerable room for manoeuvre.

The one other difference, although less clearly related to values, is the greater range of activities found in voluntary organisations responding to our survey, when compared to private or not-for-profit organisations. However, this may change as the latter are encouraged by government to diversify.

The influence of the public sector

If we found it difficult to draw a line between the voluntary and private sectors, it also became clear that many organisations had a strong statutory stake in them. These included: a private care company with a contract to manage two local authority homes, where the authority still owned and maintained the buildings; a not-for-profit trust where management was a three-way arrangement between an NHS trust, the not-for-profit and a private home owner who managed the non-professional staff; and minority ethnic community centres in area C with staff seconded from the local authority. Others had been set up by statutory organisations or workers. These included: two not-for-profit companies 'floated off' from statutory authorities; a co-operative for people using psychiatric services; a self-help group for parents of children with learning difficulties, now transformed into a community home; and an organisation for older people, set up by statutory workers who were still at the core of the organisation both as volunteers and on the management committee. Another significant influence was the number of people with public sector backgrounds and training who worked in the voluntary and private sectors. In the voluntary sector, several organisations had representatives of local or health authorities on their management boards. A councillor chaired a local branch of a county-wide voluntary organisation. Some statutory workers 'moonlighted' as care workers in private home care agencies or volunteered in their spare time.

A significant element of funding came from statutory authorities. Even in the private sector, three-quarters of those surveyed relied on benefits for part of their income.

Statutory workers also worked within voluntary and private homes – speech therapy was one example we encountered – although this may stop as costing systems get tighter. We also found that they worked alongside non-statutory agencies: for example, one of the private home care agencies in our study put carers in alongside statutory services for clients in need of support. A service user there said: 'Even though one's private and one's social services, it doesn't make any difference to them or us.'

Given these strong links, it is not surprising to find that public sector values were diffused throughout the independent sectors. Whether this will continue into the longer term, however, is open to question. As professionals are dispersed through a wider variety of organisations, fewer will have a public sector background. Links between the sectors may lose their richness as they become confined to monitoring and letting contracts rather than the broader support functions that local authority voluntary liaison officers, for example, have carried out, and as divisions are hardened between purchasing and providing roles.

Finally, several of our case study organisations – including some from the private sector – stressed that they should not substitute for the statutory sector, whom they saw as having the central responsibility to ensure that care was provided to those who needed it.

4
Ways of organising

Voluntary and private organisations are expected to bring flexibility and responsiveness to the consumer into community care. This chapter examines where responsibility lay within the different organisations in the study as well as the ways in which they organised themselves. It then explores how far these forms of organisation allow for the flexibility and responsiveness that is expected of them. Finally, it looks at the links between organisations and their importance in a total pattern of community care.

Management culture

We found the following 'ways of organising' in the agencies we studied.

Top-down

Charismatic (a leader with a vision, to whom the organisation defers)   A crucial starting point for many organisations had been the charismatic founder, who was able to collect a network of people and commitment around his or her entrepreneurial vision. A day centre for elderly people, a local medical charity which now runs residential and nursing homes, a national charity which provides a range of services to disabled people, a community organisation for minority ethnic women and several private agencies all started this way. In some cases, the influence extended many years beyond the founder's death. This does not always mean that the founder retained the dominant influence. In two organisations we studied, charismatic founders maintained their involvement but successfully handed control over to a broader group of people.

Hierarchical (with clear responsibilities at different levels of the organisation) This culture, with power and authority clearly residing at the top of the hierarchy, could be found in the more complex organisations. Based in what have traditionally been accepted as models of good practice in both public and private sectors, this way of organising was often expected by funders and other collaborators, as the next chapter will demonstrate. It was seen as inherently rational and was resisted by those who felt that care and support could not be routinised.

New managerialist (decentralised but with strategy, budget levels and standards dictated from the centre) Current management thinking was encouraging a more decentralised approach, where local or project managers had a great deal more autonomy when it came to day-to-day running than in traditional structures. However, although the rhetoric talked of devolution, authority in organisations which came into this category still clearly lay at the centre and moves to become more 'business-like' seemed also to be associated with the need for more control from above. Thus, strategy and financial decisions still came from the top as did codes of practice and quality guidelines (although these were sometimes worked out in consultation with staff).

Bottom-up

Participative management (co-operative decision-making, informality, personal contact) Work and communication was managed on a face-to-face basis, with mechanisms for giving all those involved clear access to decision-making: 'We make decisions after as wide a consultation as possible, even though it slows down decisions' (user-based advocacy group).

Where there were staff in participative organisations, they worked closely with membership and management and saw their direction as coming from them. There was a resistance to anyone assuming a clear leadership role. Where there was more than one member of staff, the staff were typically organised on a collective basis and distinctions between paid and unpaid staff were not rigid. Structures were usually flat; values and codes of practice were often implicit rather than explicit. Individual workers, paid and unpaid, sometimes had a lot of autonomy, either because they were trusted or because they were under an obligation to operate within clearly shared and stated values.

A participative mode of operation does not necessarily imply that an organisation is amateurish. Some participative organisations had developed carefully constructed procedures to ensure that members were fully involved in decision-making: 'Everything needs to be written down and efficient so that everyone knows what's going on'. In this minority ethnic women's organisation, while the worker was responsible for day-to-day management, management committee members were always around helping to run the organisation.

Devolved, federal This differed from a hierarchy or new managerial approach in that strategic and policy decisions were taken by the member bodies rather than the parent, which operated as an umbrella, providing information, training and other resources to branches or member organisations, campaigning for the cause and conferring a seal of approval. The only sanction that the parent had in these cases was the threat to withdraw its name along with the status and protection that this implies. Branches in these organisations could remain fairly small and face-to-face but enjoy some of the advantages of economies of scale, and the credibility of a larger organisation. One local branch only survived because the national umbrella was prepared to put money into it to tide it over a difficult period. However, some respondents in our study saw this way of organising as too loose a structure, allowing amateurism and territorialism.

Charismatic and participative management cultures were easier to sustain in smaller, simpler organisations. Hierarchy was likely to develop as organisations grew and responsibilities needed to be clarified and more clearly allocated. Participative management was particularly likely to be found in community and user organisations, although it also applied to some family businesses and small donor organisations: the counselling agency mentioned above, for example, or a small voluntary day care centre.

Exactly half of the donor organisations in the study were branches of a larger organisation compared with only 15 per cent of private organisations. In larger organisations, genuine devolved management was most likely to be found in donor organisations. The few corporate care firms we studied in detail were more likely to be part of a new managerialist organisation or even of a more traditional hierarchy. This was also true of the few not-for-profit organisations. Most user and community organisations were 'stand-alone' organisations.

Where does the buck stop?

Even where small enterprises operated according to participative values, it was generally much easier in the private sector to see 'where the buck stopped' than in other types of organisation. Indeed, in one case, the participative ethos actually inhibited staff from making any critical views known to the owner. They didn't want to upset the atmosphere of everyone working together like a family.

It was often less easy to identify a particular person in charge of user and community organisations. Those we studied resisted vesting authority in one person, because that would threaten their collective ethos. Nonetheless, most were still very clear about where the buck stopped, i.e. with their members/users. They were also very clear about their membership criteria, compared to donor organisations. Where staff were employed or where there were people from other backgrounds in the management committees, there was a strong commitment to ensuring that ultimate control lay with the users or community representatives. While two organisations commented on the imbalance in practice between knowledgeable staff and less experienced members of management committees, in another it was quite clear that the staff were not in control and felt unable to exert the influence they would have liked.

Donor organisations (and some community organisations) were typically trying to balance a wider range of accountability: to funders, trustees, donors, managers, users, carers and relatives, the community, staff, members and volunteers. In many, even the concept of membership was loose: they tended to be open to 'anyone who is interested'. In some organisations, management committees tried to mediate between different interests – a role which did not always combine well with the need to make strategic decisions. Sometimes this meant that the staff had the real power, even if trustees 'carried the can'. On the other hand, some respondents from the private sector felt that the voluntary sector was committee-bound and that inexperienced volunteer managers did not give staff enough autonomy, a view echoed by at least one worker in the community sector. But while it has inherent pitfalls, this multiple accountability can, handled effectively, give a range of people the opportunity to get involved in running, and influencing the policy of, local services.

In smaller donor or user organisations, the fact that management falls on one person may be less to do with culture than the fact that there is no-one else to take over. In one organisation the same management committee member had been running the organisation for 25 years. Dependence on one person, for whatever reason, can leave the organisation very vulnerable. In the case of a sports club for disabled people, it was doubtful whether the club would survive if the person running it lost interest or was unable to carry on. He was already into his 80s.

Flexible?

Many of the organisations we studied did feel that they were able to be much more flexible and accessible than the statutory sector. In local government, said one respondent, 'the attitude is: it can't be done'. A community organisation said they would not be able to have the lunch club organiser doing fifteen hours a week outreach if she was employed by the local authority. Public sector services were seen to be particularly restricted in relation to what kinds of home care they offered and when it was available. Part of the reason given for this was the sheer size of public bureaucracies; a worker in a home for people with learning difficulties pointed out that it was much easier to change policies in an organisation employing five staff. Another reason was the increasingly tight budget constraints within which local and health authorities operated. A private home care organiser said that: 'Xshire was the best in the country until the government took exception to it'.

Whereas local authorities are increasingly constrained in the use of their resources, independent organisations have the flexibility to raise resources from donors and the private market. The use of volunteers and self-employed workers respectively is another source of flexibility, although some felt that under financial pressure it could become exploitative – one volunteer started delivering meals-on-wheels with her baby in the back of the car. But this difference can be overstated; statutory services do use volunteers themselves, while private and voluntary organisations have their own sources of inflexibility. Some private sector entrepreneurs said that they didn't feel they would be able to achieve what they wanted to do in the voluntary sector because there were 'too many committees'. At the same time the need to keep beds filled to break even or to charge for extra services was a source of inflexibility in the private sector.

Voluntary organisations are sometimes characterised as 'amateurish'. But management in all sectors sometimes took place 'by default' – no-one had thought of doing things any other way. Many organisations described the way they were run as 'loose but getting tighter'. Nonetheless, one manager who had come from the private sector and was trying to pull his donor organisation into the twentieth century found the voluntary sector 'so woolly – it's good at talking, not doing'. He described a time in his organisation when there was no director and 'any one of four committee members might be telling them what to do'. In other organisations, a lot was based on trust – that volunteers were: 'right-minded people', or that, 'whoever

was in the right place at the right time' would take responsibility. This looseness can offer workers and volunteers
considerable space to exercise initiative. But it can just as
easily silt up, be unsupportive and let opportunities pass
by. One user organisation felt that it was good at dealing
with crises but not in establishing the procedures that prevent the crises.

Many small and medium-sized organisations, from
whatever sector, had very little core capacity. Structures
were flat, not by design, but because organisations had
inherited a very low administrative core and tight running
costs.

> One local agency manager was responsible for 16 staff
> and found himself doing everything from mending
> the boiler to development and fundraising work.
> Another organisation which was involved in coun-
> selling and training for a growing client group had as
> its co-ordinator a part-time worker with her own case-
> load.

This has major implications for the capacity of smaller
organisations to take on contracts or adapt to new opportunities.

Close to the consumer?

Among donor organisations, larger and more professional
organisations were more likely to develop formal user
involvement policies than smaller volunteer-run organisations – many housing associations responding to our questionnaire, for example, had developed a whole range of
user involvement policies from charters and quality circles
to representation on committees. They were more likely to
involve users on committees, although not always success-

fully – in one organisation, meetings tended to be at a time the users could not make and little attention was given to the question of how an inexperienced user could be supported to make a full contribution to a committee full of professionals. Private organisations were slightly less likely to have formal user involvement mechanisms and, by the very nature of their composition, did not offer the option of involving users in management through committee membership.

Smaller donor organisations were also less likely to have formal user involvement mechanisms than their larger counterparts. But while user control or involvement can take place in the spaces within loosely organised agencies, it can be put on a firmer basis if there are clear procedures and expectations built into an organisation's structure. Even in user or community organisations it was sometimes difficult to ensure that users had control. A worker in a user organisation with two local authority professionals on a management committee made up mainly of users still felt that the professionals dominated too much. On the other hand, professionals in three organisations felt that volunteers and carers in their organisations had been wary of giving more responsibility to users and that this had only happened when professionals had become involved.

Networks

What became increasingly clear during our study was that it is often difficult to define clearly the boundaries between one organisation and another. This was especially true of donor, user and community organisations. Small organisations go outside their boundaries for resources that are available within a larger organisation. One single-person agency we visited worked closely with other similar one-person projects to provide a network of services to the locality that would not have been possible if each had worked alone. In our study localities, consortia involving people from across the sectors had set up donor and community organisations. One of our case study agencies had been set up by a local voluntary sector development agency to which it still had links. As we have seen, management committees were often networks in their own right. One black community leader we interviewed said that often it was the same people who got involved in different initiatives and that the line between public sector professionals and the voluntary sector was very blurred in his community. This was not surprising in communities where there was still a considerable gap between need and organisational capacity.

One respondent thought smaller organisations were more linked into the local community because: 'Big organisations look to their own maintenance too much'. Generally, voluntary organisations of all types in our study had wider networks than private organisations and were more likely to co-operate with other agencies. But there were exceptions, especially where private sector managers had previous voluntary or statutory experience. The private sector may be discovering the benefits of co-operation.

Voluntary organisations of all types were more likely to belong to formal federations or to come together in temporary campaigning alliances. However, a growing number of private organisations (a third in our sample) had joined federations for the support and information and the implicit or explicit seal of approval given. Examples include the UK Home Care Association (which covers voluntary and private organisations) and the National Care Homes Association. These federations are also concerned with promoting the private sector in a community care market which is still slightly suspicious of them. They are unlikely to be involved in campaigning or public education on behalf of users. What this means for purchasers and service users is that independent agencies cannot be seen in a vacuum.

What they can deliver and the values they espouse are often very dependent on their relationship both with other independent organisations and with statutory bodies. But such networks also ensure that independent organisations are more 'transparent' to each other and in some sense accountable across their own boundaries.

5
Pressures for change

So far, we have described the variety of organisations which already go to make up a 'mixed economy of care'. We have suggested that distinctions between user- and community-based organisations and organisations that provide services for others on the one hand, and between different degrees of complexity on the other, may be as important as distinctions between for- and non-profit organisations in making sense of this mixed economy. By 'making sense' we mean understanding why providers enter the care market, what they are trying to do there, how they manage themselves and what they offer the service user. We have also suggested that the range of organisations on offer needs to be seen as an interdependent network rather than as a set of competing alternatives – a network in which the statutory sector still plays a crucial role, including as a provider.

What pressures do these different organisations face in the current policy environment? And what implications do these have for their ability to continue to contribute to a diverse economy of care? Organisations in our study raised concerns about the effects of regulation, monitoring and quality standards and the formalisation that these required. They questioned the suitability of ideas about management that were sweeping across their territory. They were feeling the pressures of financial restraints in the face of increasing demand, and for some the new market meant expand or die.

Organisations are not entirely creatures of their environment. Pressures for change also came from internal imperatives. But wherever these pressures come from, it seemed to us that they often push organisations to become more like each other rather than to remain distinctive. If current policy seeks to create a welfare mix that involves a variety of providers, action will need to be taken to develop and sustain that variety.

Regulation and monitoring

In the past, some organisations felt that there had been remarkably little regulation or monitoring from statutory funders. The move to a contracting culture had brought with it a renewed emphasis upon regulation and monitoring. Most organisations agreed that external control and regulation was increasing. The managing director of a private home commented:

> *If I had a magic wand, I'd go back to 1986 . . . Then the Home Leader's responsibility was the welfare of the resident. Now he or she would spend all of the working week at a desk filling forms in. The actual caring is secondary to regulations.*

National and European Union regulations that affected organisations in our study related to the preparation of food, health and safety, lifting, fire regulations, environmental health, registered homes legislation and so on. Many organisations had introduced staff training on food hygiene and handling or carried out refurbishment of kitchens to get them up to the new standards.

Many residential organisations – from both private and

voluntary sectors – were very aware of the need to provide a safe environment and found inspections helpful. Home care organisations, where there are no mandatory registration or inspection requirements, were keen to 'be seen to be monitored and to be operating satisfactorily'. Several of those in our study were members of the United Kingdom Home Care Association (UKHCA) and felt that its guidance and recommended procedures gave them a credibility with purchasers that they would not otherwise have.

Home owners or managers were very aware that failure to implement regulations could lead to them being closed down and some were wary of criticising inspectors' judgements. However, some regulations were felt to be inappropriate and inflexible. Fire and other safety regulations often had the effect of conflicting with the principle of providing an ordinary home for people. For example, whilst information about complaints procedures for people living in residential homes is vital, having a notice displayed in the entrance hall of a home does not necessarily do anything to create a culture where complaining is acceptable, but can make it less inviting or homely.

> A woman with profound learning disabilities in one private home lost her purpose in life after being told that she could no longer sit in the kitchen with staff. To her, the kitchen was the centre of the home's life, as in many families. Elderly residents in another home wanted to keep their doors open as it made them feel less isolated. But fire regulations meant that this was out of the question.

There were examples where regulations had been applied inconsistently by different statutory authorities or by different inspectors.

One private residential home for elderly people had carried out costly renovation work in order to increase standards only to be told by a subsequent registration officer that the improvements were not adequate. The home owners had taken out a loan over a four-year period at some considerable cost.

No-one criticised the costs of implementing regulations which were seen to be appropriate. But regulations bear a disproportionate cost for small agencies, whose budgets are tight. The owner of the home where residents wanted to keep their doors open was thinking of spending £6000 to install a new kind of door in a new home – a substantial sum for a voluntary organisation.

Health authorities and social services departments have a difficult task. They are handing over public money to private and voluntary providers over whom they have imperfect knowledge or control. Furthermore, rules and regulations are necessary in a world where not all providers can be relied upon to put the interests of service users first. One reaction may be the attempt to control through ever-increasing regulation:

> *It is as though protective regulation were governed by a ratchet mechanism that allows it to move upward but never, or at least, infrequently and only by small degrees, downward.* (Bardach, 1989)

The balance between safeguarding residents and allowing a level of risk-taking commensurate with life in the community is extremely delicate. But it is impossible to control every eventuality from a distance. The middle manager of a housing association commented that: 'It only takes one thing to happen in a social services department to start a rule that goes country-wide.'

If regulations are not to push everyone into the same mould, they need to be context-specific and take into account differences in both providers and consumers. There should be scope for users to decide what level of risk they are willing to accept, something which currently seems to be entirely missing.

Regulations also need to allow for the use of volunteers. One local group for the elderly asked ruefully how older people, who had been preparing food all their lives, were likely to respond to demands that they should attend a training course. Another organisation was no longer able to provide meals cooked locally by volunteers because of regulations. A small local donor organisation pointed out that: 'using volunteers means you run on goodwill and you can't force people to do things'.

Quality

Many organisations in our study were considering or already implementing quality systems. In a climate of severe financial restraint, where organisations are competing to obtain contracts with purchasers, evidence of 'quality' policies may give an organisation an edge – at least until everyone else has caught up. For other organisations, quality initiatives stemmed primarily from a desire to improve services for users.

British Standard 5750, as an externally validated quality assurance system, was particularly popular, if expensive. The director of a national donor organisation said that BS 5750 was important for a federal organisation because it helped them pick up problems in outlying branches. But BS 5750 is about consistency and systems rather than outcomes. Several people asked what quality standards actually said about an organisation, other than that it had followed a particular quality course or module.

Community care services rely heavily on relationships between people and involve many intangibles which are difficult to measure. We would argue that a quality service is marked as much by what makes it stand out from the rest as by its conformity with common standards.

Quality standards were criticised in some organisations as being top-down and imposed by management. They did not address the concerns of service users and carers or encourage ownership by the whole staff group.

> One voluntary residential home which brought external consultants in to implement a quality module found the report extremely unhelpful – the author appeared to have little experience of residential care. In another organisation, professional standards dictated from above were causing grave concern to local staff, who were being told not to reveal anything about their personal life to their service users.

Staff are essential to quality services and a number of organisations in our study were developing staff training such as National Vocational Qualifications (NVQ). Several thought that they would be seen more favourably by purchasers if they could demonstrate that they had a high-quality service and workforce. Purchasers in our study and elsewhere specified what proportion of staff need to be qualified and to what level in their discussion with providers over contracts. However, few organisations saw qualifications as an essential for incoming staff. They were looking for personal caring qualities, the 'right' attitude or previous experience in the field. One home owner said she preferred to train her own staff than have them ready-trained.

Some organisations were developing their own training. For example, a counselling centre was working through a standards, ethics and accreditation scheme to get their training accredited. For user and community organisations whose principal concern is to provide an employment opportunity for service users or local people, accreditation is an obvious channel to follow. However, few of them had the resources to put into training, either in the form of spare time or money.

Training staff is generally an investment larger providers are prepared to make, but it fell heavily on small agencies, especially if their staff then moved on and they had to train up someone new. It also reduced contact time with clients in small organisations which could not call upon training officers to organise this for them.

There was little evidence that purchasers were willing to pay the cost of developing quality or training programmes. Indeed, in one of the study authorities, an umbrella organisation which had received public funds to provide training to small voluntary organisations had its application for joint finance turned down because training was seen to be the responsibility of the service provider.

Tightening up on management

Getting staff qualified through NVQ was only part of the drive to become more 'professional' – a need which organisations from all parts of our organisational map expressed. One organisation saw its ability to expand as dependent upon developing sufficient management expertise; another which had already been awarded contracts was worried that this success might 'overtake' them, if they did not develop the management expertise to match.

Many organisations had reviewed their operations either on their own initiative or at the behest of funders, often through the use of external consultants. In several large 'donor' organisations, new directors were brought in to bring the organisation into more professional shape: one was described as being in 'the quill pen era'. Here, where there had been serious financial difficulties in the past, the new director argued that an organisation with such a large turnover could not be left to 'the efforts of middle class women with nothing much else to do'. In two organisations, the 'old guard' on the management committee had been encouraged to resign and make way for new members.

Sometimes the need for change was defined from outside, for example, by the need to win or retain a contract: this stimulated one organisation to introduce employment contracts for staff, to have regular staff appraisal to ensure that they did 'not dress too scruffily' and above all to be more professional. Elsewhere the need for change was defined internally – by management committees or part-time co-ordinators who saw the writing on the wall, or parent bodies who were tightening up on the procedures they expected of their branches. The spotlight put on the liabilities of trustees of national organisations under the recent Charities Act and by contracts is forcing national organisations more generally to reconsider how autonomous they are prepared to allow local branches to be.

> The director of one national charity commented that 'the charming elements of total autonomy are impractical in the tough world of competition'. This charity had more than a hundred homes and services – all with different ways of collecting and presenting information and with several different accounting periods. The organisation was 'moving away from the introspective belief that because we have a lovely founder, all will be well' and recognising 'that we will have to change in order to survive'.

Housing associations had already felt the wind of change. The Housing Corporation demanded a more professional approach of the housing association in our study in the late 1980s. It saw the association as amateur because many staff came from the voluntary sector rather than having professional qualifications. But tenants were critical: 'We got what we wanted from volunteers, now it's more bureaucratic – there are a lot of people with titles in the organisation'. It was not only users who felt they'd lost out. An area manager in the same organisation thought they'd lost their 'gut feeling – it's instinct versus rules'. The local organisation is trying to remain flexible – for example, in its admission procedures – but this is getting more difficult. In another organisation, a local pop-in centre for older people was being asked by its umbrella organisation to adopt 'proper audited accounts'. But they felt this was excessive for an organisation which dealt with so little money.

At the same time as autonomy for some managers was being reduced, people who had moved from the statutory sector to independent or 'floated-off' agencies found their autonomy had increased. One manager found he had more freedom to use initiative, even if the results of doing so were highly visible and immediately available to senior managers through computerised systems. It is possible that, once systems have been established in other organisations, and the organisation is run the way that new managers want, more autonomy will be given to local managers there.

In line with the new managerialist thinking, greater devolution was often recommended to hierarchical organisations by consultants. Others, as we have seen, saw the advance of highly specified guidelines and standards from above as the advance of a new kind of bureaucracy. Even though they accepted the need for clear boundaries within which to operate, huge files of directives and procedures from the centre seemed to contradict messages about autonomy.

In the end, opinions about more 'professional' management were divided. Community and user organisations often get their 'street cred' precisely because they are informal and accessible. They may lose their ability to act as confidantes and advocates for people if they become too 'professional'. On the other hand, one carer we interviewed said that she had more confidence in the organisation that was offering her support because it now had 'professional people at the top'.

Business culture

Added to the need to become more 'professional' was the advance of the business culture across the caring field. Some voluntary sector managers were being sent to a local business school for training or encouraged to take an MBA. Others talked of the need to be more business-like and the director of one donor organisation described himself as a businessman.

One of the most important elements of business culture is to be one step ahead of competitors. Owners of at least three of the private agencies in our study were members of local care home consortia. One of them commented that, although in the past home owners would not even tell each other their bed vacancy rates, they were now prepared to share this information. However, he also saw the consortia meetings as a way of getting information about how he could be that little bit better than other homes.

Business culture also stresses the need to market and promote the organisation. In the contract culture, as one large charity said, you have to go out and sell your services.

A 'floated-off' trust commissioned a PR firm to help market itself and produced a newsletter and a glossy brochure; a housing association had just changed its name and was 'getting into presentation and house styles'; a branch of a national home care agency had monthly regional marketing meetings, had developed a new logo and 'turned itself inside out'.

This emphasis on image, however, is a surface change. It may even make it harder to see what is really going on underneath. As a carer said of a home her father had previously lived in: 'The salesmanship all went by the board' once he moved in. The manager of a donor organisation also said that promoting themselves in a way which increases the chances of contracts being awarded might result in their organisation losing its distinctiveness and ending up like a professionally managed local authority unit.

Organisations were also being pressed to develop business plans with clear targets when applying for funds from the local authority and to have accurate accounting and costing procedures.

> The organisation that was described earlier as being in the 'quill pen era' had just bought a computer and a volunteer accountant was setting up systems for them. A large national charity was getting to grips with the need to synchronise information on its homes and services and has spent thousands on computerisation.

The need to look carefully at unit costs was encouraging voluntary organisations to account more closely and plan more carefully, but the business culture was seen to take a very short-term and quantitative view of costs. Indeed, closer accounting in statutory authorities was affecting the support in kind that organisations could get from this quarter in the form of transport, advice and premises.

A local society for people with a physical disability

said that it was no longer possible to get help easily: 'everywhere you go there is a charge'. They wanted to put on a holiday playscheme but the school where they wanted to hold it was no longer able to provide the facilities free of charge because of LMS (financial devolution to school governors).

There was much readiness in the voluntary sector to learn from commercial ways of operating. But there was also a recognition that the messages that are currently being purveyed under this banner are not always appropriate. Indeed, the business culture that is sweeping through the public welfare field does not necessarily reflect the most up-to-date business thinking, which is now showing more interest in staff motivation, trust, co-operation and social goals – areas in which the voluntary sector has much to offer. As Leat (1993b) argues, it would be ironic if the voluntary and community sectors were to abandon some of the practices on which leading thinkers in the private sector are now drawing.

Resources

Two further problems were identified with a more business-like approach. One was the cost in time and money to organisations of setting up more and more systems; the other was the impact on committed volunteers and managers. There is rarely any money to support the increasing administrative case-load that 'more professional' management, service agreements and contracts entailed. One director commented: 'We can't provide a service unless it is well-managed, otherwise it will fray round the edges. But funders will only pay for face-to-face work.' It was widely reported that getting money to cover core costs, which include training as well as administration and management, was 'almost impossible'.

One user organisation was given three and a half per cent to cover core costs as it was assumed, erroneously, that they already had an adequate infrastructure. One day care contract for £66,000 p.a. over three years made no allowance for administrative or management costs, which were expected to be met through charitable donations. Another contract for domiciliary care in a sparsely populated rural area included no allowance for staff travel.

Furthermore, if funding is on a year-to-year basis, or contracts are delayed, key personnel and experience can be lost as staff seek a more certain future elsewhere.

Late payment by authorities, who fail to realise the tight margins on which many independent agencies operate, is a particular problem: we were told of one home care agency which went bankrupt because of this. Another one had instructed a debt collection agency to recover their unpaid fees from a local authority.

New and pioneering organisations often find themselves particularly hard-pressed. One minority ethnic organisation for people with mental health problems found its one paid staff member in constant demand for consultations with other agencies and public authorities. While the high profile for their concerns is welcome, these demands limit the time available for face-to-face work.

Another problem for organisations who have a participative management culture is that the increase in paperwork changes the way in which managers work and reduces job satisfaction. We have seen that a number of managers wanted to remain 'hands-on'. Staff and users in their organisations often preferred to see the manager working amongst them. But as Lewis (1993) has pointed out, the new managerial culture can involve so much more administration that managers lose contact with front-line staff, volunteers and service users.

Volunteers whose commitment is to face-to-face work do not want to be absorbed in administration. One commented: 'I need to be working with people. I hate committees'. Carers in one organisation which had several contracts felt that it was moving away from its roots, that it had become more technical and less fun to be involved with. As a result volunteer commitment had reduced.

Volunteers are not, as government expectations sometimes suggest, a homogeneous group. Flexibility is needed to allow for different skills, time constraints and levels of commitment. In a number of caring organisations, organisers felt they were there as much to help volunteers as service users. In other organisations, including user organisations, volunteers carried a considerable amount of responsibility for complex tasks. Indeed, a number of paid staff started out as volunteers.

Several organisations reported difficulty in recruiting volunteers. If new pressures lead to a further loss of volunteers, voluntary organisations will lose their ability to be responsive. Some felt that the Charities Act had made it more difficult to show appreciation for voluntary effort.

One woman running a small lunch club said that volunteers now had to buy their own meals and that she could not even buy a volunteer a bunch of flowers from the organisation's grant. She would have liked to have had some money to say thank you to them.

Loss of volunteers can also lead to a reduction in flexibility.

One organisation, now that it is being awarded contracts, no longer needs fundraising efforts from volunteers. But if it were to lose its contract, this organisation would find it difficult to gear itself back up to being a primarily volunteer/fundraising organisation.

An important feature of all types of voluntary organisation is the voluntary nature of their management committees or boards. Many people spoke of the growing difficulties of getting management committee members: 'We're scratching around to get people to serve.' New demands – whether from the community care reforms, more general tightening of standards or a sudden awareness of their responsibilities as a result of the new Charity Law – meant that some people had resigned. The new Charity Law led to some anxiety among management committee members in user organisations, wondering whether they might be ineligible – because they might have debts on record or because of periods in a psychiatric hospital.

Often contract conditions require new skills of management committee members in marketing or developing a business plan. In some organisations paid workers were training existing management committees to be more aware of their responsibilities and to be more formal in their conduct. There was rarely sufficient time or money available to give volunteers adequate training, particularly for the new responsibilities arising out of the reforms.

Many of the larger, more 'professional' organisations were trying to encourage people with backgrounds in business, banking, accountancy and the law to become members of management committees or trustees.

A counselling organisation was thinking of trying to attract people with business skills but commented upon the difficulty of finding people who also had knowledge and interest in counselling, adding that they were counsellors not managers.

In some organisations, finance and general purposes committees involving people with 'business' or 'professional' skills had been set up, which met more frequently than the full committee or board of trustees. Less experienced management group members found themselves on subcommittees dealing with fundraising and social events while the new guard got on with the real business.

It is, of course, essential that trustees have the expertise to carry out their responsibilities, but this creates problems for organisations who see it as part of their role to involve users or people from the community who have not had this sort of experience before. Less experienced members of committees often feel left out.

> Carers in one organisation said that they did not understand the new and complicated language of contracting and felt that it was inevitable that they would be edged out, particularly as most management committee members were health or social services professionals able to negotiate their way through this world with ease. They said they needed time and space to assimilate service specifications.

Either some way needs to be found of bridging this gap between the different groupings involved in voluntary organisations or we need to question definitions of 'professionally run' and allow the space to involve people with different competencies.

Funding

Many respondents were worried that finance for the voluntary sector will increasingly be channelled through contracts or fees for service. Several saw the future of funding for organisations which fail to secure contracts or who do not wish to become involved in contracting as uncertain. If this happens, what will be the fate of organisations who are not in the market for service contracts or who wish to continue to provide the complementary services which they developed against a background of mainstream provision? As one director with some success at fundraising said: 'How many funding sources are there out there?'

One area where there is still new money is in advocacy. In one of our localities, advocacy was already well-supported, but in the other two, new funds had been made available for advocacy and consumer forums. However, many voluntary organisations who combine an advocacy role with a service provision role are worried that this will no longer be possible if government funding is increasingly tied to service contracts. One advocacy organisation had decided against taking statutory funds – it felt it would be compromised and needed to be outside the system to retain any power to challenge.

But even those organisations whose main income is from contracts or fees can find themselves in difficulties, bearing the costs of a transfer of service which is taking place against a background of severe cost constraint. Several organisations talked about funding being cut at the same time as the work involved in acquiring or retaining funds from the statutory authorities was increasing. Sometimes funding difficulties are passed on to the consumer.

> One voluntary organisation had set its rates above what the local authority would pay and was 'topping up' out of the personal allowances of residents who had no funds other than state benefits.

One donor organisation providing residential care was expected by its authority to fundraise to meet the acknowledged shortfall in funds. In other instances funding constraints were being passed on to staff.

One of the directors of a private sector organisation

said: 'The big risk is to descend into using slave labour'. Workers within that organisation had lower rates of pay than in the statutory sector and no unsocial hours allowance.

This situation was replicated in some of the other private sector organisations studied. Some used self-employed staff and did not give holiday pay.

There was evidence that the transfer of services in some authorities had led to reduced terms and conditions for staff. Work elsewhere has suggested that some statutory authorities are seeking to keep their costs down by offering voluntary organisations substantially less than that spent by the local authority on a similar service (Lewis, 1993).

In one authority which had put its residential care services out to tender, staff had been sacked from the local authority and had to re-apply for their old jobs a few weeks later with the private company which won the contract. The residential social work post was abolished and the wages of the care assistants reduced. A 'floated-off' trust had retained enhanced pay and conditions for existing staff but reduced them for new staff. The director of a large donor organisation was considering whether staff pay and conditions might have to be reduced if, as seemed likely, purchasers were not going to increase fee levels. A matron in one of their homes had already taken a voluntary pay cut so that funds could be available to hire a qualified member of staff.

The continuity and morale of staff is likely to suffer with a knock-on effect on quality and continuity of care.

Expansion and diversification

Standards, quality, new managerialism, growth and for-malisation, business cultures and financial pressures – all these pressures drive organisations to formalise and per-haps to become more alike. Smaller organisations – those run by one or two people or pursuing a participative approach to management – seemed to stand the most chance of maintaining their distinctiveness, if they could survive financially. But contracts were felt to favour larger organisations, who have the expertise to bid, who are a known quantity and who can afford to carry initial losses. Smaller organisations felt they might well go to the wall unless there are alternative sources of funds or unless they expand and formalise. There was general concern that small private residential homes would not survive the shake-out that was following the reforms and that 'once the big boys get in' the same would apply to home care too.

Providing residential or nursing home care on existing fee levels was a problem for many organisations. Some were receiving top-ups from their local health authority, including one 'floated-off' organisation which was also fundraising from private trusts. Some owners of small homes said it was more difficult to accept DSS residents in a smaller home because there were fewer residents to sub-sidise the person on benefit. Others felt that small homes were only viable as part of a larger organisation which could cross-subsidise from larger homes. In one organisa-tion these loss-making 'smaller' homes had 16 and 30-plus beds respectively. Other small home proprietors were building extensions in order to remain viable or tap new opportunities – a move dictated by the market but surely counter to the intention of de-institutionalisation?

Small homes may run the danger of becoming isolated and inward-looking, but they offer more chance of a homely environment. In one home with five residents, staff came to say goodbye individually to each person at the end of their shift. Obviously this would become impossible if the number of residents increased significantly.

In order to stimulate the market in domiciliary care provision, central government is encouraging independent residential care providers to diversify.

> One large voluntary residential care agency wanted to diversify to meet the increasing need, as they saw it, for a spiritually-based service. A private home believed that without diversification it would not remain competitive *vis à vis* the corporate sector. Its owners were planning to move into terminal care and day care.

Private home care providers in our study were critical of some aspects of diversification. They pointed out that managing and monitoring home care, which takes place out of sight of the managing agency in people's own homes, is quite different from managing residential care. There was some evidence that workers with experience in institutions found it difficult to adapt to smaller community homes or home care.

A number of voluntary organisations already have considerable experience of diversification. They have been doing it for years as new needs arise and have a lot of experience to offer. But the need for diversification is currently framed in terms of assuring the viability of a business and the desire to add to existing competitive advantage. One of the authors of the Department of Health guidelines on diversification has recently spoken in terms of 'protecting the flow of residents for the future' by providing them with home care now so that they will hopefully purchase residential care later (Whittingham, 1993). As such, diversification raises the spectre of growing cradle-to-grave 'Big Brother' service empires which will replace the more diverse networks of care that users currently draw on and could even move into the business of merger and takeover. How far will these empires provide choice and individual care? And how will they be different from the local authority service empires of the past?

Much that is happening to independent organisations at present is seen as a result of government policies. But the pressure for growth does not come only from outside. As one respondent said: 'If you stand still, you wither and die' – something which seemed to be happening to two of the organisations in our study (see Taylor, Langan and Hoggett, 1994). But, as organisations grow, so the pressure grows on them to move from a small, simple organisation to a larger, more complex form. This may be because of an increase in demand; the acquisition of more staff (paid or unpaid); getting a grant or a contract; acquiring premises; a significant increase in membership; or an increase in activities or area covered. We have suggested that, as an organisation grows so management gets separated from operations, membership (in voluntary organisations) and service users. But is this inevitable? Is it possible to grow without losing co-operative ways of working and the relative autonomy of staff, or the power of members to influence the direction of the organisation?

Many of the small and medium-sized organisations we spoke to found themselves at a watershed. Some were at the point where they felt a face-to-face way of working was no longer possible. Several had consciously decided to stay the size that they were and had turned down opportunities to take on more staff or projects. One had separated from its parent to become, in effect, a franchise – a word used by another to describe its relationship with its branches and a form that others were also considering (see also Norton and Temperley, 1992). Networks, as we have seen, allowed others to survive as smaller organisations. Still others were considering appointing directors or co-ordinators but were concerned about changing power relations (let alone where to get the money from!). Was it possible to have a co-ordinator without power settling around that person?

Schumacher is famous for his argument that small is beautiful. But his argument is more to do with finding simple ways of managing complex tasks. Many organisations in the changing community care environment are struggling with just that challenge. Little will have been achieved by the reforms if one set of large service empires is replaced by another which does not even have the democratic accountability of the public sector. There is an urgent need for debate and exchange of experience on alternative ways of organising and investment to back it up – franchise, co-operatives, coalitions and networks – and to engage with those at the forefront of commercial management thinking in an exchange which recognises the value of voluntary as well as business management.

6
Conclusions and recommendations

The concept of distinct public, private and voluntary sectors is becoming more and more inadequate to describe the range of organisations now operating in the community care field and the relationships between them. Developments over recent years have created what one US commentator calls a 'fuzzy and ill-defined territory between public and private which needs to be understood . . . if we are to design social policy effectively' (Rein, 1989). This study suggests that it is a complex territory with hybrid organisational forms, overlaps in personnel and values, and where the services provided often depend on relationships between different players in this new institutional environment. But it also suggests that the diversity it contains may be under threat.

Why is diversity important?
Research suggests that 'The designation of an organisation as public or private, its relationship to government, and its sources of funding are not the critical variables in determining how effectively it responds to people in trouble' (Bush, 1988). As another writer comments, 'in service delivery, *how* may be more important than *who*' (Kramer, 1994). Users may be more concerned about their right to a service

than where it comes from (Gray 1993; Wilson, 1993), a finding confirmed by the service users with whom we discussed our findings. So why *is* diversity important?

A diverse range of consumers will have diverse needs and preferences. An older Muslim woman, for example, may need day care; any provider could in theory meet this need, but not necessarily in a way that she could use. Her gender, class, ethnicity, religion and life history will add a dimension of 'requirements' which dictate how her needs can be met.

> One of the agencies we studied provided a lunch club for older Muslim women, where they were able to converse with each other and with staff in their own language about experiences that were understood and shared, and where their diet met the requirements of their religion. To offer one of these women a service in a community centre where it was impossible for her to eat the food her religion requires or to make the necessary religious observances would not meet her needs. Nor would a setting where men were present, where no-one spoke her language or had any understanding of her traditions.

Such requirements are not an optional extra. But service users may then have preferences which, though not essential, would lead them to choose one provider over another if choice was available.

Secondly, diversity allows services to develop which are 'close to the consumer'. Services that are locally-based or that are provided by people from the same ethnic community, for example, may be easier to approach and easier to use. Some people find it easier to use services which are 'among friends and close to home'.

A third reason for diversity is the need to draw on the

widest possible range of resources and energies in meeting
need. This means providing different ways for people to
become involved in provision and support in the community – as volunteers, as entrepreneurs, as trustees or managers, as fundraisers, as paid staff, as members of a self-
help group.

A fourth reason for diversity is the need to develop new
ways of doing things, to have the potential for risk-taking
and experiment. There is no one right way of delivering
care. The capacity needs to be available to try out new
approaches.

Current policies advocate competition to encourage
responsiveness and efficiency. But competition alone does
not necessarily produce variety, as is clear from other fields
of activity, where competitors all flock to copy a successful
model or politicians scramble for the average voter. It is also
important to recognise that diversity does not guarantee
individual choice: that depends on service users being given
the right to a service and control of the decisions about the
service which they will receive. It also depends on purchasers understanding what service users want and need.

There are many pressures which, without intending to,
could reduce this diversity and wash away many of the
'grey areas' that have in the past allowed for informal net-
working, flexibility, resourcefulness and the generation of
new ideas in independent organisations. Community care
is a risky business. Lord Keynes once said that: 'It is better
to be roughly right than exactly wrong.' In creating a competitive market in community care and trying to minimise
risk, it is important that current reforms do not drive out
the commitment of donors, volunteers, service users and
entrepreneurs to a diverse range of activities, and the informality and responsiveness to expressed need that they contribute.

So how can purchasers and policy makers maintain and

develop this diversity and the range of energies and values that it releases? In this concluding chapter, we make some practical recommendations based on the findings of our study, and we raise a number of questions that need to be debated further if diversity is to be maintained – suggesting some possible models to support future provision.

Recommendations

Local and health authorities

1. Know your independent sectors   There is already a 'mixed economy' of care in most areas. Chapter Two described what to look out for and what it offers. This, along with an understanding of what service users need, should be the foundation for any new policies. Authorities need to take steps to develop a clear up-to-date picture of who operates in their area, what they do, how they operate and, most importantly, where they fit into local patterns of provision. Although many authorities have been developing a much improved picture of what exists through the joint planning process over the past three years, this information needs to be available to staff and members throughout both local and health authorities.

2. Invest in development and infrastructure   If a diversity of provision is to be maintained and developed, an investment needs to be made in market or community development, to support new and emerging organisations, especially minority ethnic organisations. In this role, local government should also be providing research and intelligence to stimulate and develop new forms of production and organisation that can cope with the increased demand of the future. There are examples from abroad, such as social co-operatives in Italy.

Organisations need support through change or growth. Core and development funding is essential to their ability to respond to new needs and demands. This may be in-house; it may also be in the form of funds for accredited consultants; or it may be through umbrella organisations, which also provide individual organisations with a forum for making their voice heard with purchasers. If funds are only allocated for direct service provision then short-term cost savings may be gained at the expense of the continued viability of the organisation.

3. Invest in variety Purchasing arrangements should be designed to allow small organisations access to contract funding and service agreements, to encourage consortia bids and to build-in some security for organisations who do not have the capacity to absorb financial risk. Purchasing patterns should be kept under review to ensure they do not exclude small and minority ethnic providers.

This investment needs also to recognise and support the patchwork of 'taken-for-granted' services and activities in which mainstream services are embedded and without which there would be much greater demand. These are unlikely in the present climate to be priorities for contracts, but are an essential part of total provision.

Pluralism in delivery requires pluralism in funding. A balance needs to be maintained between contracts and service agreements on the one hand, where the authority defines the service to be offered, and more flexible funding arrangements, which allow for different definitions of need and new ways of delivering services.

4. Invest in advocacy Diversity alone does not give people a choice. In the field of community care, many choices are made under pressure, through intermediary purchasers (care managers or doctors) and from a limited selection.

Service users are rarely then in a position to keep chopping and changing until they find the service that suits them best. Even if this were possible, continuity of care is an important aspect of quality and their best interests are unlikely to be served by constant change. For all these reasons, service users need access to independent information, advocacy and mutual support.

The development of advocacy services in one of our localities has allowed users to have a say not only in public but also in private sector provision, and offers models for building-in quality, to which we shall return later in this chapter.

Resources are also necessary if requirements for consultation with independent and user organisations are to have any force. Consultation works best when it draws on a strong base of involvement which has developed over time and when it has the resources to be well-informed and communicate widely.

Some authorities see consultation with potential suppliers as prejudicing planning. To see the voluntary sector in particular solely as a pool of suppliers in a market is to ignore the dual role which many have played in both supplying services and drawing on that experience to influence policy. Whether private or voluntary, independent organisations between them have a fund of knowledge on the way in which need has been and can be met in local areas, which can contribute considerably to the development of knowledge in purchasing and planning authorities.

5. Do not overregulate   Choice and diversity will not develop if purchasers regulate every aspect of the service they put out to tender. It is tempting, especially in an age when litigation is becoming more common, to insure through regulation against risk. But caring is a risky business. If the Audit Commission finds it difficult to come up with meaningful performance indicators for community care, we can be sure that there are aspects of this business which cannot be predetermined and measured but have to rely on trust. Overspecification and overregulation will undermine the development of independent organisations. They will simply create pale imitations of public sector services.

There is a danger that public sector service empires will be replaced by regulation empires. Purchasers should avoid this and seek instead to build up support for good practice, through inspections which emphasise education and development rather than control and through investment in training. Regulations and standards should also take account of the standards that users of that service wish to see. Nothing we found suggested that all regulation should be abandoned, but some of the resources that are now going into regulatory structures could usefully be diverted into support for user- and carer-based organisations to help them define the standards and quality of support they need.

6. Recognise the importance of networks Organisations do not operate in isolation; an emphasis on competition and unit costs could discourage links between organisations. Statutory funding policies should guard against this and be prepared to put resources into independent networks, which can act as nurseries for new organisations, provide the infrastructure smaller organisations need and encourage organisations of all sizes to work together. They should also recognise the importance of the support in kind which public sector workers have given to independent organisations, both informally and formally, and ensure that new systems of public sector management leave the space for workers to continue to play this role.

Implications for central government

1. Long-term investment   Most of the above recommenda-tions have significant cost implications. Our political sys-tem does not encourage governments to take a long-term view of spending. But the prospect of increased demand in the future requires a longer-term view in the field of com-munity care. We believe that the investment that diversity requires is a positive investment for the future and will pay for itself by reducing future crises, and by reducing turnover of staff and organisations in a service which requires continuity.

Some social services departments will be affected by local government reorganisation over the coming years. Many voluntary organisations fear that this will mean fur-ther cuts in already tight budgets and that services defined by outsiders as non-essential will be the first to go. It could also affect the development of constructive partnerships between statutory and non-statutory organisations. Ways need to be found of minimising the risk this presents to local patterns of care.

2. Public sector provision   A true mixed economy implies voluntary, private and statutory providers. Although few people would wish to see a return to the monopolies of the past, many of our organisations wanted to see a continued, if more limited, role for public authorities in 'hands-on' provision, and not a residual one which would turn the public sector into a stigmatised and underfunded last resort.

3. Charity law   If resources are to be released for the future, the tax privileges offered by charitable status need to be used to optimum benefit. Charity law needs to ensure that organisations are properly managed and publicly accountable while maintaining the tax incentive for people to put resources into care.

At one end of the scale, Gutch (1992) has suggested the creation of a 'socially responsible business' which would include private businesses engaged in social enterprise as well as voluntary organisations engaged in commercial enterprise and attract a level of tax exemption lower than that of the 'pure non-profit' but still capable of attracting investment. At the other end of the scale, charity law should recognise the public benefit of many service user-based organisations and allow user-based organisations in the welfare field to specify a majority of users on their management committees and yet still enjoy charitable tax privileges.

Other problems that charity law needs to address are the burden currently carried by trustees which, at a time when government is trying to encourage local management of a variety of services and facilities, is reducing the pool from which managers can be drawn.

Finally, charity law needs to address the issue of the relationship between national charities and their branches in a way which allows for the support and credibility of a national organisation to be combined with local flexibility.

Questions to be addressed

These recommendations have focused on the implications of our study for policy makers and purchasers. But they highlight a number of issues in the current provision of community care for which no easy solution is available, and which need to be brought to the centre of debates about community care if diversity is to be maintained. The following key questions need to be addressed by purchasers, policy makers, voluntary and private organisations alike:

How can voluntary and private organisations maintain the strengths of 'simplicity' as they grow: responsiveness, face-to-face communication, informality and flexibility?
In asking this question, we are not wishing to promote an unquestioning 'small is beautiful' approach. Small is not beautiful when organisations are isolated from new developments, unsupported and struggling to survive. But there is a need for innovative new models to preserve the advantages of simplicity and autonomy and yet provide for organisational growth and economies of scale. This is an issue which has attracted the attention of some of the foremost thinkers in the business world for some years, but if it is to be relevant across the independent sectors it needs to draw together ideas and experience across the sector boundaries. More research, more sharing of experience and ideas is needed to evaluate, develop or adapt organisational forms: to explore the potential of franchising and similar models; to develop loose network models which are light on their feet – capable of giving support without becoming bureaucratic; and to evaluate the different national/ local structures that voluntary organisations have evolved over the years. Larger organisations in the sector could have an increasing role to play in supporting smaller and user-based organisations and need to consider how they can best do this.

How can high-quality care and support be achieved without overstandardisation? Are the same standards necessary for all kinds of organisation?
Government has set up a deregulation task force to try and reduce the amount of unnecessary regulation. Our study suggests that there is considerable support for regulation as such. It is its implementation which is causing the headaches.

Quality is an extremely difficult thing to define in relation to care (Leat 1993b). Ways need to be found of defining quality standards from below rather than imposing them from above. We have suggested in the body of this book that the existence of networks and joint working arrangements which include the statutory sector makes organisations more visible. Positive and open working relationships between organisations in the future may be one way of spreading good practice and spotting danger points before they become a crisis.

Beyond this, one proposed solution is to privatise regulatory agencies, with groups of licensed regulators competing on the open market for custom. But this would run the danger of 'regulator capture': regulators and providers could easily form cosy alliances with the user bearing the cost.

The solution currently favoured by local authorities seems to be to set up working groups of professionals, representatives of various interest groups and, occasionally, carers and users to come up with a regulatory framework. The danger is that by attempting to please everyone, the groups would please no-one and yet remain unchallenged because of the investment in consultation that has already taken place. It is also likely that professionals would still dominate many of the groups and there is still nothing then to stop the framework being imposed inflexibly across the field whatever the size and capacity of the agency.

A third model would be based on the proposition that the problem of regulation only arises because users of services do not have an adequate voice and someone has to protect their interests. If users were adequately organised and empowered, the facilities they use would be forced by pressure from below to adapt services to their requirements. Under such a system, regulation would be context-specific. A general framework would be devised by government but as a guide rather than a set of prescriptions. The support to allow service users to refine this to their requirements could be provided by user-based advocacy projects with access to users across all sectors.

How can user, volunteer and community involvement be maintained when the task of management is becoming more sophisticated and the liabilities more onerous?

Current government reforms across the welfare field are seeking to involve more and more people in managing public services – local management of schools is the obvious example. But where are all these managers and governors to come from? If they are to come from the communities and constituencies that use services, every attempt needs to be made to encourage rather than discourage involvement. Apart from the provision of resources for training and support, this may mean considering different levels of liability for different levels of involvement. It is likely to mean waiving some restrictions on who can be involved in management and trusteeship if users and ex-users of some services are to become involved. It may also mean more flexibility around availability-for-work regulations for those on benefit, so that people who are unemployed do not lose benefit when they volunteer.

How can forms of audit and accounting be developed which take into account the longer-term and social costs involved in community care?

If the transfer of service provision results in costs being driven down, the long-term effect could well be high staff turnover, low morale and poor-quality services. It is difficult to talk of community care solely in terms of the market and individual consumption. Community care is a 'public good'. Although better accounting systems can undoubtedly improve its quality and reduce waste, they cannot alone guarantee an effective service. More consideration needs to be given to long-term costs and definitions of quality.

Future models of care

Many commentators have remarked on the major cultural change which will be required if public authorities are to become 'enabling' authorities. But 'enabling' can mean a variety of different things. At one end of the spectrum is a minimal model whereby the purchasing authority meets simply to let contracts and where the role of the State is that of ensuring that the barriers to a free market are removed. Our study has suggested the need for a much wider role with the capacity to:

- invest in community and enterprise development;
- invest in independent support services for small non-statutory organisations in the locality;
- allocate grants (not contracts) for innovative projects: i.e. providing new services, providing services in new ways, providing to new groups;
- develop the infrastructure to allow users, carers and providers a meaningful voice in the joint planning and commissioning of services, and encourage public debate on community care priorities;
- allocate grants to independent advocacy projects (and require contracted providers to introduce advocacy in their own services);
- develop frameworks and structures for user-led and context-specific regulation.

Not all these functions would be performed within public authorities. Public authorities need to respect the autonomy of independent organisations and support the development of independent support and advice. But the likely rise in demand for support to enable people to live a full life in the community is going to require imagination, resources and a willingness to listen to what service users really want. It is going to need more than an increase in the number of organisations competing to provide the same services. If patterns of provision and support are to be developed which provide diversity and choice for service users, government – central and local – needs to play an active role in supporting and investing in that diversity.

Appendix A
Methods

The study was based in three localities (see Appendix B) and involved two phases:

- mapping
- case studies.

The mapping phase involved:

- interviews with local umbrella organisations and other key local informants
- a postal survey.

Interviews with key informants gave us an overall picture of the range of private and voluntary organisations operating in each sector, which we used to build a list of organisations known to be providing community care. We then sent questionnaires to a sample of 600 of these organisations (200 in each locality). The sample was selected, not on a random basis, but in order to ensure coverage of the range of organisations we expected to find: private and voluntary; with or without government funding; residential and non-residential. We also ensured that a quota of minority ethnic organisations, housing associations and umbrella bodies were included. The questionnaire sought basic information on:

- age of organisation
- aims and activities
- coverage
- affiliation
- constitution
- membership
- management committee structure
- staffing (paid and unpaid)
- budget and sources of funding
- user involvement.

In both the interviews and the questionnaire, we also asked about the effects of recent policies in the community care field.

Information from the questionnaire survey is summarised in Appendix D. Because of the way the sample was selected it does not offer a representative picture overall, but does allow comparison between different types of organisation.

The information gathered in the mapping phase was used to develop an organisational map based on ownership and size (see Fig. 1, page 9) and to choose 33 organisations from across this map to study in more detail (see Appendix C). These were mainly selected from the sample, but where there were gaps we approached organisations suggested by our preliminary interviews with key informants.

This case study phase gathered qualitative information on:

- organisational roots and values
- management culture and structure
- the effects of recent policies, including in the community care field
- perceived differences between the sectors

- contact and collaboration with other agencies
- involvement of users and carers
- key management pressures.

We carried out a minimum of two long interviews in each organisation with a manager or the owner on the one hand and a service user, volunteer or a member of the front-line staff on the other.

Four organisations were then interviewed in greater detail, with up to 15 interviews carried out in each case. Our choice of the four in-depth case studies again reflected the dimensions of ownership and size but was also based on ambiguities or changes in these dimensions:

- a user-based organisation which was facing the challenge of growth;
- a donor organisation with a strong statutory input;
- a donor organisation undergoing major changes to become more business-like;
- a private sector organisation with one director who had extensive experience of management in the public sector.

In two of the three localities (B and C), local panels were set up as a reference group to discuss emerging findings. These panels involved service users, carers and people working in the voluntary and private sectors.

Appendix B
The localities

The three localities where fieldwork took place were chosen to reflect very different environments, in order that we could ensure as wide a spread of organisations as possible.

	A	B	C
Political composition	New Right Conservative	Traditional Conservative	Labour
Welfare orientation	Market	Family and community	State
Geographical area	Suburban (outer London)	Rural	Urban
Population	290,600	198,800	253,230
Percentage of people from minority ethnic groups	4.7	0.005	10.7
Percentage of people over 65	17	21	19

Figure 2   Locality profile

Area A has a well-established voluntary sector which has traditionally made good the deficiencies in statutory provision. Its voluntary organisations are well-established with 33 per cent formed before 1960 (comparable figures for areas B and C are 20 per cent and less than ten per cent). A number of voluntary organisations there feel that the local authority is reneging upon its responsibilities by taking the sector's commitment for granted and consistently underspending.

Area B has no voluntary sector infrastructure. Its voluntary organisations typically receive little funding from the statutory authorities, who spend less on the voluntary sector than is the case in the other two areas. Voluntary organisations tend to be small-scale, isolated, heavily dependent on volunteer effort and dispersed across a large geographical area with extremely poor transport links. As a result organisations have found it more difficult than in the other areas to network and develop a dialogue with the statutory sector, although this is developing fast.

Area C is one of the highest per capita spenders in England and Wales on social services, with the local authority still the principal provider of community care (Department of Health, 1993). However, the city and county councils have actively developed and funded voluntary and community organisations. The area has an active voluntary sector, with many community-based organisations, a strong self-help movement and a range of umbrella organisations. This is reflected in the greater confidence of its voluntary sector to criticise the statutory sector without fear that funding or relationships will suffer.

Areas A and B are more interested than Area C in divesting themselves of their in-house services. Area A's social services department is keen on contracting out as many services as possible and much of its in-house services has been 'floated off' into the private sector. Area B created a not-for-profit trust to which it has transferred the majority of its residential provision. Both areas have a well-developed private residential and nursing home sector. Due to the reforms, the private home association in Area B is now enjoying better relationships with the social services department. Area C is generally more suspicious of private agencies than the other two areas, but its health authorities have supported the development of private homes for people leaving psychiatric services.

Area C has the most substantial minority ethnic population of the three, with people mainly of Afro-Caribbean or Asian origin (both Indian and Pakistani). Traditional services, whether statutory or voluntary, have been criticised for not meeting minority ethnic needs. Voluntary organisations are developing fast in the minority ethnic communities, with community centres often staffed by workers seconded from the County Council. However, specialist community care organisations for minority ethnic groups are only now developing. Despite their numbers in Area A, we found little evidence of minority ethnic organisations there.

Local and health authorities in all three areas have established networks and forums with users, carers and the voluntary sector and some appear to be genuinely trying to incorporate these various perspectives. However, uncertainty and frustration were expressed in all three areas about how committed the statutory authorities really were to making a success of consultation.

Appendix C
The 33 case study organisations

The case studies are listed according to their place on the organisational map. Precise classification is impossible – as we have said in the main text, it is a fluid model and organisations change. However, within each category we have, as far as possible, listed organisations in order of size and complexity. Organisations are also classified as they appeared when we chose them. Some we discovered to have a strong statutory stake in that they were staffed or part-owned by a statutory organisation. These have been marked with an asterisk. Branches of regional or national organisations are particularly difficult to place, especially since in each case we interviewed people from the larger body as well as the branch. Those which are judged to be autonomous or semi-autonomous are marked with two asterisks.

Small/simple user organisations
1. A pioneering and radical group of non-disabled people and of people with learning disabilities. The project aims to foster and encourage independence for people with learning disabilities through advocacy, enterprise and active citizenship. Its activities include training, speakers, workshops and consultancy. Values are equality (everyone

involved is a co-worker), user involvement and community development.

2.   **Locally-based branch of a carers organisation. The only one in the area to be set up by a carer rather than the social services department. Its values are to provide activities and support that carers want. The programme of activities is therefore member-led. Involved in consultation over the community care plan but little optimism that carers' needs will be met, because of insufficient resources.

3.   *A therapeutic earnings workshop scheme set up as a co-operative by the manager of a health authority psychiatric day centre. Currently supported by a worker from the social services department and at a critical point in its life as it has few members and is seen as lacking dynamism and somewhat exclusive. Difficult to classify: it was originally chosen as an example of a user-led co-operative, but considered not to be one, since it clearly has a strong statutory stake in that its survival depends on the worker.

Small/simple donor organisations

4.   Small bowling club for elderly people with visual impairment. Meets during the bowling season only. Receives funding from donations. Membership is declining due to age of members and the impossibility of getting regular transport from local agencies.

5.   **Small locally-based club for older people, with many older people deriving satisfaction from being volunteers at the club themselves. Relies mainly on donations. One small informal part of a larger local organisation which is providing services under contract. It is part of a federal organisation which it finds useful for insurance purposes.

6.   Christian Good Neighbours Scheme started by local ecumenical council members. Many of the scheme's volunteers are active Christians and sit on the council. Provides transport, befriending, shopping, etc. for elderly and housebound people. Publicises widely but has more volunteers than it can use. The values are Christian ones of helping your neighbour, including those worse off than yourself. Relies on informal networks to vouch for volunteers.

7.   Black mental health organisation set up in the last few years. Has one worker only so the range of activities possible is limited. It is considering getting involved in housing and homelessness and also wants to expand to provide more services. Values are to try and address the needs of Afro-Caribbean people who feel they are badly served within the mental health system.

8.   A semi-autonomous short-term project under the umbrella of a Council for Voluntary Service, but with its own premises and advisory group. Set up to develop services for carers. Its one worker is trying, with a lot of energy, to develop networks and put tangible initiatives on the ground within a very short time-span. Works closely with other agencies and aims to be led by what carers see as important. Development and support are key words.

9.   **Small organisation for carers and people with cerebral palsy. Started in the 1970s but membership is declining now. Has a part-time support worker but nowhere for people to meet as a group. Well linked into local consultative forums. Finds it a strain to have to provide surveys of need before they can get any funding for services. Recent partnership with housing association.

Small/simple private organisations

10.   Small private home care agency having great diffi-culty in surviving. Owner's values are love of elderly people rather than making a profit. Deriving a great deal of support from the UKHCA (United Kingdom Home Care Association).

11.   Christian private residential home. Small number of residents (five) and owner thinking about expanding to 10–15 to survive. Keeping a Christian faith is very impor-tant. Family-run with joint owners working virtually non-stop because of size of home. Caring staff but staffing levels leave little time for activities with residents.

12.   A private home care agency set up by doctors seven years ago for people discharged from hospital. The co-ordinator has a background in the statutory and voluntary sectors and continues to work closely with the public sec-tor. She is now going independent as a franchise and con-sidering appointing a worker to join herself and the administrator. The organisation belongs to UKHCA and its ethos is to provide a professional service which provides choice, respects the customer and maintains people in the community.

Medium-sized user organisation

13.   Umbrella mental health users' advocacy group set up in 1988 incorporating three elements, each with paid work-ers: self-advocacy through patients councils, citizen advo-cacy and individual patients advocacy. Run with a large number of volunteers who are actively involved at all lev-els within the organisation, including on the management committee. Most of those involved are psychiatric system

survivors. The values are advocacy and user empower-ment and this is encouraged through open participatory management structures. Debate about whether to become more professional and appoint a co-ordinator.

Medium-sized community organisations

14.   Community centre set up by local minority ethnic women some twenty years ago. Activities include advice, education and training and running a lunch club. In the last two years, it has appointed two part-time staff members. Strong sense of solidarity of involvement and still very much run by local women (the founder is still involved). Looking to expand its activities.

15.   *Community centre for people from minority ethnic groups dating from late 1970s. Managed by a worker sec-onded from the local authority but accountable to the cen-tre management committee who are in charge of what happens. Social services fund the care services including the luncheon club and meals-on-wheels facilities. The cen-tre is composed of sub-groups reflecting different ethnic groups as well as clubs for women and elderly people.

Medium-sized donor organisations

16.   Care group set up 25 years ago by an energetic local volunteer who is now its President. Raised the money to build its own day centre with a work centre attached that does contract work for local industry. Four staff, lots of vol-unteers and an atmosphere of energy and bustle. Caring,

love and commitment are key words. Talked of possibly setting up another centre.

17.   Voluntary residential home for adults with learning disabilities (none with severe disabilities) set up by parents with support of the local and health authorities. The manager has a health authority background. The management committee, which now includes a resident, has changed. Only three parents remain on it. Strong developmental normalisation ethos with independence a key word. Tries hard to be resident-centred.

18.   Independent housing project established in 1983 providing accommodation for people with learning disabilities. Founded by parents but staff have become increasingly important stakeholders. The management committee has changed in composition and has more professionals on it, particularly business people. Staff feel ambiguous about what is expected of them and there are strong pressures for the organisation to adopt a more business-like and formalised way of operating.

19.   Originally part of the Family Welfare Association, this counselling centre changed its name in the 1970s to reflect the work it was doing, providing counselling for emotional and personal problems and training counsellors. It runs largely on volunteer and trainee resources, with four staff plus administrative support. Professional and participatory ethos but run by a part-time co-ordinator who has her own case-load and feels that organisation is at the boundaries of its current capacity. Recently appointed a fundraiser.

20.   **Autonomous branch of a national organisation providing support for carers of people with Alzheimer's

Disease (ADS) and day and weekend care to people with ADS under contract. Inextricably linked with the local statutory multi-disciplinary team who provide many of the management committee members. Well poised to be awarded further contracts. Values are dignity and respect for carers and people with ADS.

21.   *The voluntary arm of an organisation which incorporates a statutory side – both working within the drugs and alcohol field. The statutory side refer people on for longer-term support than they are able to provide. The director has a health authority background and shares a vision with his counterpart in the statutory arm of having a partnership. Some tension over roles, accused by some of wanting to make the volunteers too professional.

22.   A traditional voluntary organisation, with a long history, for older people. After a period of problems and drift a new director has recently come in from the private health care sector. The organisation has a number of projects and affiliated branches supported by its development officers – which are fairly autonomous, in keeping with the federal structure adopted by the national organisation to which it is affiliated. Culture has been fairly amateurish in the past, but present director brought in to change that. Caring and service ethos. Affiliated to a national charity.

Medium-sized private organisations

23.   A private nursing home bought by its present owners fairly recently; had been losing money under its previous owners. They already run a private clinic. They have brought in an administrator with a background in private industry and a matron from the NHS. Strong caring ethos.

The managing directors are consultants who are looking to expand.

24.   Private residential home poised to expand and diversify into caring for other people besides the elderly. Young joint-owner who grew up in the business. Believes that competing with the corporate care companies is the only way to survive. Recently scoured out the old guard of staff, appointed matron who shared his values. Introducing NVQ, wants to apply for BS 5750, formulating care standards.

25.   Recently established, purpose-built, medium-sized home for people with severe learning difficulties. Set up by three managing directors, one of whom has a health authority background. Saw a need for accommodation that wasn't being met by existing facilities. Neither of the other two directors are from the public sector. The organisation has another home and plans to expand further into semi-independent living schemes and respite care. Caring and normalisation are key words. Management is approachable, staff at all levels feel that their opinions are listened to. Many staff are from the public sector.

Large donor organisations

26.   Local Christian voluntary organisation modernising but trying to retain important elements of its tradition including its mission to help the poor. Originally set up by a female doctor at the beginning of the century. Entrepreneurial in its first 60 years and set up residential homes and health services. Hiatus for next 30 years. Key elements in the last two years have been entrepreneurialism, professionalism and 'moving into the 21st century'.

Over the past couple of years there have been more trustees with professional or business backgrounds and more are male. The first male director in the organisation's history has recently been appointed.

27.   **County branch of national organisation. It has a very large volunteer force and is in the process of drawing up a contract with the local social services department. Recent fundamental review with organisation opting for greater devolution. Clear boundaries within which volunteers operate and well-established system of supporting and training them.

28.   **Domiciliary care branch of a national voluntary organisation with a contract with the local authority. The national headquarters are reviewing the operations of the services and homes and seeking to improve information systems, accounting and costing procedures. This represents a reduction in autonomy for individual homes and services. Attempting to 'be more business-like without being a business'.

Large not-for-profit organisations

29.   **An area branch of a national housing association, formed in 1974, which provides group homes for people with mental health problems. It grew out of a theological discussion group which was looking for something practical to do. The area office covers two counties and 18 projects. There are six group homes in the area covered by our study. The area office is informal and participatory, but more detailed management systems have been introduced nationally over recent years in response to changes prompted by Housing Corporation recommendations.

Values are concerned with support, independence, dignity and respect.

30.   *A company limited by guarantee and a registered charity which sees itself as a not-for-profit organisation. A hybrid set up by the health authority to provide and develop accommodation for people in mental handicap and psychiatric hospitals moving into the community. Is now independent of the local voluntary organisation that lent its name to the venture in order to access DSS benefits. Some tension between the local Mental Health Trust providing clinical staff over who is in charge, who is legally responsible for services, etc. Values are about normalisation although some of the clinical staff have more institutional views.

31.   *A hybrid – a not-for-profit trust established to 'float off' the majority of the local authority residential provision within one of the study areas. Has an appointed Board of Directors and senior staff generally have public sector backgrounds. Has a business-like approach in terms of setting up systems to ensure accurate management information. More autonomy for home managers within clear boundaries. Transferred staff retained the enhanced conditions and rates of pay they had received in the local authority. New staff have lower rates of pay.

Large private organisations

32.   **Part of a corporate care company which includes domiciliary care and nursing amongst its portfolio. Has recently had fundamental review, new uniforms, logo, etc. to make it more competitive. Regular marketing meetings are held and its prime aim is to make a profit. However,

care is taken by branch manager to screen out potential workers to ensure that they are not more interested in what they can earn than in caring.

33.   **A large corporate care company which recently took over two local authority residential homes. Key words are providing what people want in the manner of a hotel rather than the previous ethos of enabling. Residential social work posts were abolished in the changeover and care staff re-applying for their old jobs received a substantial salary cut. Communication and decision-making has been improved by the move out of local authority control.

Appendix D
The questionnaire survey

Size of non-statutory sector

In this research we did not set out to conduct an exhaustive survey of voluntary and private sector organisations engaged in community care in our three case study localities. We therefore have no accurate information regarding the size of this sector in the areas that we studied. Such an analysis is complicated by the fact that many organisations, such as community associations and village halls, provide a range of services besides community care. All we can reliably say by way of the size of the non-statutory sector is that in the three areas we covered we had no difficulty in sampling 200 organisations in each area, the large majority of whom concentrated solely or largely upon providing services which could be defined as 'community care'.

Our research is based upon questionnaire survey and case study data drawn from this original sample. 253 organisations completed the questionnaire. Profiles of the different types of organisation on our 'map' are given in the text.

Age profile of voluntary and private organisations

Our survey would suggest some clear differences in the age

profile of different types of organisations. Whereas half of our sample of voluntary organisations had been formed since 1979 nearly 80 per cent of the private sector organisations had been formed since that date. Not surprisingly smaller organisations (irrespective of whether they were private day care, donor or user) tended to have a younger age profile. This suggests a much higher degree of turnover, i.e. of births and deaths, than for larger donor or private organisations. Voluntary residential homes have the oldest age profile: in our sample almost as many were formed before 1960 as after 1979. This contrasts strongly with privately-run nursing and residential homes, almost 80 per cent of which were founded after 1979. The other distinctive feature concerning age relates to the housing associations in our sample – nearly 80 per cent of those in our sample were formed during the period 1960–79.

Activities engaged in/services provided

Over half of our sample of voluntary organisations provided leisure, social or day care activities and almost a third provided support and counselling. On the other hand only one in 14 claimed to engage in campaigning or lobbying. User organisations focus very strongly on leisure and social activities and providing support. Simple donor organisations focus even more strongly on providing leisure and social activities typically by running clubs *for* people with disabilities, severe learning difficulties, etc. Complex donor organisations, by which we mean the larger, more formalised ones who may employ staff of their own, are the only kind which appear to engage in the full range of care activities. Not surprisingly, some of the gaps in voluntary provision appear to be compensated for by private pro-

vision, for our sample of non-residential private organisations focused almost exclusively upon providing home
care and home nursing.

Client group

More than one in six organisations in the voluntary sector
provided services to people with learning difficulties or
experiencing mental distress, while nearly one in four provided services to people with physical disabilities and one
in three to elderly people. In contrast private sector organisations focused much more strongly upon providing services to elderly people rather than other client groups. On
the other hand only three organisations in our sample
offered services to those with AIDS/HIV. Different types of
organisation appeared to work with different client groups
– simple donor organisations worked with the elderly, user
groups were most frequently organised by those with
physical disabilities or chronic illness. Interestingly, most of
the simple donor organisations we visited that provided
care for elderly people were actually run by elderly people
themselves, though they didn't define themselves as user
or self-help groups.

Communities served

Over half of our sample of voluntary organisations operated within the immediate neighbourhood or locality. The
local focus was strongest for simple donor organisations
and weakest for housing associations, most of which were
regionally based. Only six organisations mentioned that
they provided services specifically for ethnic minority communities and they were all located in area C – however, we
do know of at least one other organisation, a luncheon club,
catering for the needs of black people in area A. Just three

organisations specifically provided services to women only, and one only to men.

Organisational characteristics

Whereas 85 per cent of our sample of private sector organisations were 'stand-alone' organisations exactly half of the voluntary sector organisations were branches of, or parts of, a larger organisation. This was most pronounced for user groups. However, being attached to a larger organisation did not in any way appear to undermine the autonomy of most of the groups in our survey, for organisations like Age Concern or MIND were reported to operate in a loose, decentralised way. About one-third of the private sector agencies in the sample were affiliated to federations of proprietors.

Ownership and management

Different organisations prefer different ways of constituting themselves. User organisations were the most likely to have no formal constitution whatsoever (12 out of 40); on the other hand almost half of them (17 out of 30) were registered as charitable trusts. Seven out of ten simple donor organisations were registered as charitable trusts, a slightly higher proportion than complex donor organisations, a quarter of which were registered as limited companies. Just over half of the housing associations were registered as Industrial and Provident Societies.

Five out of every seven of our sample of voluntary sector organisations said that they had a membership. However, the nature of the membership differed. Whereas in user organisations it was typically limited to users/carers, for other organisations it was often open to 'whoever comes along' or defined in terms of a person's commitment to the objectives of the organisation.

A strikingly high number, all but two of the 185 voluntary sector organisations responding to our questionnaire, had a management committee or belonged to a larger organisation that had one. Whereas user and simple donor organisations recruit to their management committees primarily by election (though this often involves a lot of arm-twisting and 'volunteering') the other voluntary sector organisations recruited by a combination of election, appointment, co-option and invitation. As a consequence, the latter organisations are the most likely to have professionals and representatives from other non-statutory organisations on their management committees. Staff representation is not a notable feature of any type of organisation, and is most likely to be found in complex donor organisations, where it was a feature of no more than 15 per cent. Whilst user representation is a defining characteristic of the management committees of user organisations, elsewhere it was found in only one in three organisations, with simple donor organisations (one in five) and voluntary residential homes (one in seven) the least likely to have user representation.

Finally, the size of the management committee varies from one type of organisation to another. User organisations had the smallest committees (average size of ten) whereas complex donor organisations had the largest (average size 16). This was not simply a characteristic of size, for simple donor organisations tended to have larger committees than voluntary residential homes. It is also interesting to note that user organisations and housing associations display a remarkable degree of consistency in the size of management committee whereas complex donor organisations are remarkably inconsistent (in area B four had less than ten on their management committee whereas three had more than 30).

In contrast the private sector organises itself in a far simpler way as the problems of inclusion (of membership), representation and mediation (of different interests) are largely absent. Three-quarters of our sample were basically owner-managed organisations run either as family businesses or small partnerships or by individual proprietors. The latter is a particular feature of small businesses which provide home care services. These often amount to no more than a single woman (with a number of others on her books) who provides home care for a few hours a week to a small number of clients. The income derived often hardly amounts to a wage. Limited companies only feature strongly in the corporate care sector which is itself still very small. Even here the Board of Directors is typically very small (less than four members). Only in the corporate sector and some of the larger private residential and nursing homes is there a differentiation between ownership and management.

Staffing

Only 17 per cent of user organisations employed staff, compared with 80 per cent of all donor organisations and all private organisations. Three-quarters of all voluntary organisations used volunteers. More surprisingly, about one in four private organisations used volunteers to provide services and run activities such as transporting elderly residents to church, etc.

Sources and scale of funding

Approximately three-quarters of our sample of user and simple donor organisations had annual budgets of less than £5,000, derived almost entirely from donations, fundraising and subscriptions. In contrast 80 per cent of complex donor organisations had budgets greater than £25,000 the bulk of which came from grants from statutory agencies. However, this type of organisation is also the major beneficiary from donations, is heavily involved in fundraising and was the only type to include instances of successful industrial or commercial sponsorship.

References

Bardach, E. (1989) 'Social regulation as a generic policy instrument', in Salamon, L.M. (ed.) *Beyond Privatization: The Tools of Government Action*, Washington DC: Urban Institute Press

Billis, D. (1993) *Organising Public and Voluntary Agencies*, London: Routledge

Bland, R. (1993) 'Home truths', *Community Care*, 17 June

Bush, M. (1988) *Families in Distress: Public, Private and Civic Responses*, Berkeley, CA: University of California Press

Department of Health (1993) *Public Expenditure on Health and Social Services*, London: HMSO

Gray, A. (1993) 'Beyond the normalisation principle: The experience and perspectives of adults with learning difficulties living in private residential care', Ph.D. Thesis: University of Bristol

Gutch, R. (1992) *Contracting: Lessons from the USA*, London: National Council for Voluntary Organisations

Knight, B. (1993) *Voluntary Action*, London: Home Office

Kramer, R. (1994) 'Voluntary agencies and the contract culture: Dream or nightmare?', *Social Service Review*, March

Le Grand, J. and Bartlett, W. (eds) (1993) *Quasi-Markets and Social Policy*, Basingstoke: Macmillan

Leat, D. (1993a) *Managing Across Sectors: Similarities and Differences Between For-Profit and Voluntary Non-Profit Organisations*, London: City University Business School

Leat, D. (1993b) *The Development of Community Care by the Independent Sector*, London: Policy Studies Institute

Lewis, J. (1993) 'Developing the mixed economy of care: emerging issues for voluntary organisations', *Journal of Social Policy*, 22.2, pp. 173–92

Marceau, J. (1990) 'The dwarves of capitalism: The structure of production and the economic culture of the small manufacturing firm', in Redding, G. and Clegg, S. (eds) *Capitalism in Contrasting Cultures*, Berlin: de Gruyter

Maslow, A. (1943) 'A theory of human motivation', *Psychological Review*, 50, pp. 370–96

Norton, P. and Temperley, N. (1992) *Charity Franchising: A Guide to the Concept and Practice of Franchising Charitable Services*, London: Directory of Social Change

Paton, R. (1992) 'The social economy: Value-based organisations in the wider society', in Batsleer, J., Cornforth, C. and Paton, R. *Issues in Nonprofit Management*, Wokingham: Addison-Wesley

Rein, M. (1989) 'The social structure of institutions: Neither public nor private', in Kamerman, S.B. and Kahn, A.J. *Privatization and the Welfare State*, Princeton, NJ: Princeton University Press

Spear, R., Leonetti, A. and Thomas, A. (1994) *Third Sector Care*, Milton Keynes: Co-operatives Research Unit, Open University

Taylor, M. and Hoggett, P. (1994) 'Quasi-markets and the transformation of the independent sector', in Bartlett, W., Propper, C., Wilson, D. and Le Grand, J. *Quasi-Markets in Public Services: The Emerging Findings*, Bristol: School for Advanced Urban Studies

Taylor, M., Langan, J. and Hoggett, P. (1994) 'Independent organisations in community care', in Saxon-Harrold, S. and Kendall, J. *Researching the Voluntary Sector, Volume II*, Tonbridge: Charities Aid Foundation

Whittingham, P. (1993) 'Diversity in adversity', *Community*

Care, 18 November, pp. 14–15

Wilson, G. (1993) 'Users and providers: Different perspectives in community care services', *Journal of Social Policy*, 22.4, pp. 507–26